FOUNTAIN
OF TRUTH

Outsmart Hype, False Hope, and Heredity
to Recalibrate How You Age

GENIE JAMES, MMSC
WITH C.W. RANDOLPH, JR., MD

Health Communications, Inc.
Deerfield Beach, Florida

www.hcibooks.com

This book contains general advice and is not intended to be, nor should it be, used as a substitute for specific medical advice from a physician.

Library of Congress Cataloging-in-Publication Data

James, Genie.
The fountain of truth : outsmart hype, false hope, and heredity to recalibrate how
   you age / Genie James, MMSc, with C.W. Randolph Jr., MD.
   pages   cm
   ISBN 978-0-7573-1715-6 (pbk.)
   ISBN 0-7573-1715-4 (pbk.)
   ISBN 978-0-7573-1716-3 (ePub)
   ISBN 0-7573-1716-2 (ePub)
   1. Longevity—Popular works.   2. Aging—Prevention—Popular works.
3. Medical misconceptions—Miscellanea.   4. Medicine, Popular—Miscellanea.
I. Randolph, C. W. II. Title.
   RA776.75.J35 2013
   613.2—dc23

                                                                        2013004587

Publisher: Health Communications, Inc.
          3201 S.W. 15th Street
          Deerfield Beach, FL 33442-8190

Cover images ©Fotolia.com, 2013
Interior design and formatting by Lawna Patterson Oldfield

Because I want them to know now what
I wish I had known then,

this one's for the girls, especially:

Shelley

Sarah

Danika

Lulu

Ashley

Rilyn

Meghan Grace

Madelyn Hope

Bella

Olivia

Julie

Tovah

and

Girls Inc. of Jacksonville, FL, Nashville, TN
and Northwest Oregon

CONTENTS

ACKNOWLEDGMENTS

WITH GRATITUDE

M Y MOTHER, Betty Frank Sandusky Williams, always believed —and told me emphatically—that I could be and do anything I wanted. I wanted to please her, to make her proud, but for decades I waffled through more ambitions than boyfriends, never quite finding myself or purpose until my mid-thirties. Today at fifty-three, I have found my passion: writing for and speaking to women about health and aging. I am also increasingly jazzed about running a healthcare company while championing the growth of women-owned businesses. My life, my work and this book are embellished with my mother's fingerprints. I like to believe all are legacies she would relish.

Writing this book has been an especial privilege. Conversations with hundreds of women created the framework for a fresh dialogue on aging. From that platform, many busy physicians and medical researchers took time to painstakingly walk me through how emerging optimal aging science can translate into day-to-day lifestyle choices. Foremost among these game-changing healers is my husband and business partner C.W. (Randy) Randolph, Jr., MD. Heart and hats off to you, babe!

Yet this book would still be only wishful thinking had it not been for the belief and tenacity of Jill Marsal, founding partner of the Marsal Lyon Literary Agency. Then, Health Communications, Inc. (HCI)—our publisher for *From Hormone Hell to Hormone Well* and *From Belly Fat to Belly Flat*—stepped up to move my idea from concept to print. Much gratitude goes to Peter Vegso, president of HCI, for believing this book could make a difference in women's lives. Deep felt thanks also to Allison Janse, gifted editor and wise counsel, for guiding me away from the banal towards new information women need to hear now.

Kudos too to Kim Weiss, HCI's director of Communications, and Nannette Noffsinger, our media and public relations consultant. For close to a decade, Nannette has proven to be a rare blend of media coach, cheerleader and friend . . . one I would have thought out-of-my-league as she produced NBC's *Today Show* for over ten years and continues to work extensively around the world for NBC News. Thank heavens she is so down-to-earth lovely and, also, believes in this message.

Finally, my deepest gratitude goes to our medical professionals and staff of both Dr. Randolph's Ageless and Wellness Medical Center and our Natural Medicine Pharmacy. Each day your skills and commitment translate theory and academic medical science into a life-changing healing ministry for the patients we serve. You all are incredible.

PROLOGUE

A T THE SUPPOSED MIDPOINT of my life, two events forced me to internalize a duo of heart-nuking truths. The first: Laura Randolph's death. The second: my first gray pubic hair. Both snuck up on me. Both sucked.

I should have seen Laura's death coming. We were uncommon best friends, she being my husband's first wife. Nevertheless, from the very first encounter, I was enchanted by her bubbly laugh, off-cuff Nora Ephron wit, and wicked cool style. Laura struggled with a rare hybrid of ovarian cancer off and on for twenty-five years, yet her seemingly boundless tenacity buoyed hopefulness, even optimism in those who loved her. Those last months I refused to see my friend leaving us millimeter by millimeter.

The pubic hair, the *gray* pubic hair, is shallow by comparison. But that's me—both deep and shallow. I sat on the toilet completely flummoxed. I rarely wear glasses when going to the bathroom. When I do, I seldom scrutinize down there.

How long has it been there? Do I pluck? Has Randy seen it?

There was no way around these two magnitudinous facts. I was aging; someday I would die.

At some juncture in time, all of us are brought to our knees by the undeniable truths that we are no longer young and we will someday die. However, my personal come-to-Jesus moment was ironic: as chief executive officer of Dr. Randolph's Ageless and Wellness Medical Center, I had skin in the game of our culture's American-Idolish search for the latest and greatest fountain of youth. Actually, I had more than financial security and a career path invested: Dr. Randolph is my husband, Randy.

Randy's Ageless and Wellness Medical Center is internationally recognized as a center of clinical excellence in anti-aging medicine. Our medical professionals treat more than ten thousand patients each year. As CEO, information on the latest and greatest anti-aging procedures and products swamped my desk; I sorted it into one of three buckets:

- Mind-bending research written by highly credentialed physician pioneers typically housed in respected academic medical centers;
- Questionable studies written by medical researchers with financial ties to the fountain-of-youth potions they plug;
- Borderline-trashy marketing hype.

A fact: In this millennium, medical miracles have the potential to reduce our risk of chronic disease while positively impacting our long-term health, sexuality, and longevity. These radical advances are retooling the healthcare industry. What this means to you, me, our children, and generations to come is that we can increasingly get a heads-up before trouble hits.

Diagnostic tests can tell us whether or not we have heart disease, breast cancer, or Alzheimer's genes. New scanning technology displays if our brains are snappy-fit or in danger of turning to mush. Genetic blueprints sharply reveal how youthful debauchery or years of poor lifestyle choices can result in long-term damage to DNA, setting us up to age more rapidly.

More news (if you, like me, have a vain streak): The fields of cosmetic and dermatologic medicine have shifted into spheres of supreme artistry. Unlike our mothers and grandmothers, if you or I decide to have "some work" done, we are unlikely to come out from under the knife (or the end of a needle) looking like tightly pulled Saran Wrap or a squishy-cheeked Persian cat. Better yet, we have multiple options for a face-lift on a budget.

Still, this exploding anti-aging industry isn't always something to Hula-Hoop about. According to Global Industry Analysts, a 70- to 80-million-member-strong consumer base, "seeking to keep the dreaded signs of aging at bay," will push the US market for anti-aging products from about $80 billion in 2012 to more than $114 billion by 2015. Sadly, many of the glitzy antiaging products we shell out big bucks for are just plain junk; worse, some can be harmful.

When marketing gets ahead of medical science, bad things can happen. Hopes are preyed upon and wallets drained. Some supposed "fountains of youth" have been associated with serious side effects. At greatest risk for disappointment and despair: women like you and me, devastated by cottage-cheese thighs, a lengthening neck waddle, and an increasingly dry vagina—or a gray pubic hair.

There I was, overseeing a medical center called "Ageless and Wellness" while silently

> When marketing gets ahead of medical science, bad things can happen.

grappling with grief, my own fears about aging, and a growing sense of purposelessness. Then one day as I sat flipping through the latest oversized magazine crossing my desk, something shifted. The magazine's header read "The Future of Beauty and Anti-aging."

Four gorgeous twenty-something females (two in bikini tops) hovered on its cover. I cringed. Photoshopped beauty shouldn't be our standard for aging. That kind of beauty doesn't even look real. And, in fact, it *isn't* real.

> Photoshopped beauty shouldn't be our standard for aging.

I am fifty-three years old. Sure, I miss my cellulite-free rump, smoking energy, and pie-eyed ambitions, but I don't want to go back in time. Like any woman living more than two decades, I have suitcases full of sadnesses, wish-I-hads, and would-never-agains. I've lost loved ones, chose career over childbearing, and made the mistake of mixing men I love with my money. Still, each time something has gone wrong or fallen apart, I've had to learn how to make different, better choices. The decades I have lived are the reason I have increasingly grown more alive, more real.

I looked again at the magazine cover and thought, *What exactly does anti-aging mean anyway? If you aren't aging, aren't you . . . well . . . dead?* I wondered, *What if every woman could know right now what only the experience of the next two to four decades could teach? What if it were possible to glean and transfer that wisdom? What if I could facilitate a forum where women in their thirties and forties got a one-up on positive aging and living? What if I could enable women fifty, sixty, seventy, and beyond to internalize "now or never" and act accordingly? What if I could find myself again in the process?*

I made a decision to write a book that cut through the clutter and confusion surrounding this anti-aging movement. I committed to entwine new, mind-popping medical science with stories of women who are exquisitely traversing the decades. I imagined a future where this book would ignite a movement, shifting the paradigm of what it means to cultivate a more beautiful interior with age. What it means to grow *more real.*

But what is the truth about aging? How can we cut through the hype, false hope, and even the baggage of our heredity to discern a future that women can desire and even be excited about? I wrote this book to find out. By interviewing dozens of pioneering medical researchers, I discovered:

- Which medical science advances have the potential to reverse or retard aging at a cellular level;
- The clinically proven "superconditions"—for example, lifestyle choices—that most impact health, well-being, and longevity;
- How much of this emerging medical science on aging is readily accessible and actionable for the everyday woman on a budget.

I also personally interviewed hundreds of women ranging from age nineteen to ninety-three. I asked them all:

- What do you fear most about aging?
- What are your regrets?
- What excites you now?
- What are you most looking forward to?
- What is the most counterintuitive advice on aging you have to offer?

In just a few months I had a database of fabulous, make-it-happen women: women thumbing their noses at the notion that we must grow increasingly fat, dull, dried-up, and disconnected as we age; women in their twenties and thirties caught up in the debate of whether women really can have it all, all at once, or in stages; and older women considering elastic-waist jeans, plucking chin hairs, and suffering heartbreaking losses yet determinedly becoming more vital, vibrant, and relevant every decade.

Intersecting science with real-life stories spawned something special: a fresh approach to recalibrating how we age boomeranging many preconceived notions. I became increasingly excited as I researched and wrote. Then something unforeseen occurred—a collision of knee-buckling disappointments and sadness caused me to lose my sense of purpose, question the faith that has always been my compass, and avoid my face in the mirror. It took me a while to find my way back. I didn't do it alone. I needed the help of new wisdom and fresh tools. I share this with you, too—my story—from my heart to yours.

Tell me a fact and I'll learn.
Tell me a truth and I'll believe.
But tell me a story and it will live in my heart forever.
—Native American proverb

INTRODUCTION

I'M IMAGINING YOU PICKED UP THIS BOOK for one of three reasons:

1. You don't feel as vibrant as you once did. When you look in the mirror, you are not thrilled with the face and body staring back at you. The adage "You are as young as you feel" makes you nauseous.

2. You've had a wake-up call. Either you or a woman you love has had a brush with something feared—cancer, heart disease, multiple sclerosis, Alzheimer's—and you are newly motivated to do everything possible to protect your health and to live longer.

3. You are at that tipping point, probably somewhere in your thirties, when things you once took for granted in your twenties don't come easy, if they come at all: quickly losing three pounds after a weekend binge of margaritas, chips, and salsa; having enough unquestioned energy to cheerfully work, go for a run, hang out with friends, and/or cook dinner and take

care of preschoolers; wanting and having sex *all the time* to preferring an extra hour of sleep over frisky bedroom moves.

You wonder, *Is there something, anything, I can do to slow down or turn back my aging?*

Is it possible my getting older could somehow equate to my becoming better, becoming someone more *versus less as the years go by?*

My answer is a resounding "Yes!" We can't stop aging, and we shouldn't want to. But the idea that we can age differently, with greater self-reliance and ever-swelling joy, is not the wine talking—it's a medical fact.

Physically, biochemically, mentally, and sexually, women peak in our twenties, plateau in our thirties, and begin a sharp descent in our forties. According to aging expert Mark Houston, MD, *between forty and fifty is the decade of vulnerability. During these years, women age the equivalent of 18.6 years, while men age 15.2.* From fifty on, we can make choices that positively impact our health and how we age; however, the older we are, the harder and longer it takes to slow down the clock or undo damage from decades before.

From conversations with thousands of women, I have grouped the female life stages like so:

Stage 1: The Age of Arrogance

You are between twenty and thirty and you are in good shape, have high energy, think like a lightning rod, and have a sizzling sex drive. You're not particularly motivated to shake up lifestyle choices that work for you now, and you feel sorry for older women with droopy boobies, big bottoms, and lackluster lives. You are certain your future will never morph into such a cliché.

Stage 2: The Age of Reality

You are between thirty and forty. You have gained five to fifteen pounds, feel a bit sluggish, and have sex once or twice a week but fake it more than you want to admit. You wonder if you need a prescription for an antidepressant. You have started reading health magazines and following Dr. Oz on Twitter. You call your mom for advice.

Stage 3: The Age of Vulnerability

You are between forty and fifty. Everything seems to be spinning out of control: your periods, weight, hot flashes, workload, family responsibilities. You doubt yourself a little to a lot, especially when scrutinizing your reflection in the mirror. You go to doctors for help and can recite your mom's health history as if it were your own.

Stage 4: The Age of Now or Never

You are over fifty. Sure, you would like to be thinner and look younger, but something more profound has your attention: mortality, yours and that of those you love. A corner of your mind recognizes that now is your make-it-or-break-it time. If you don't thrust forward immediately to reprogram lifestyle choices, *your health and dreams* may fall away for good. You regard your mom's foibles with awakened empathy.

Whatever age you might be, sit up and take notice. *Right now* is your "Age of Opportunity," your crucial moment. While results may come easier and quicker if you are in your thirties, it is never too late to reap the benefits. My recommended approach integrates Randy's expertise in the emerging science of age-management medicine with enviable women's perspectives on "fountains of truths" as old as dirt.

Part 1 describes why lifestyle medicine, the science surrounding the cellular-level impact of everyday choices on health and hormone balance, must become your personal manifesto. The biggest variable accelerating your aging: estrogen-related belly fat. Randy and I offer hope and solutions for naturally rebalancing unhealthy hormone levels, which will allow you to lose unwanted pounds and inches once and for all.

Part 2 offers more natural tips to burn off your fat and turn back your age. Super news: What is good for your waist is also great for your face. Even better, follow my guidance and your sexual nature will transform you into a cocreative powerhouse.

Part 3 draws from conversations with hundreds of women, sharing six proven pointers for filling up and spilling over with the best your life has to offer.

PART ONE

YOUR AGE OF OPPORTUNITY

WOMEN TODAY HAVE THE OPPORTUNITY to age very differently than our mothers and grandmothers. We are no longer doomed to become increasingly fatter, sexless, and senile as hormone levels diminish and we move through and beyond menopause. Emerging science, called "lifestyle medicine," proves beyond a shadow of a doubt that daily habits influence not only how fast and well we age but whether or not our genes express health or disease, thinness or fatness, contentment or depression. More exciting, breakthrough medical research surrounding the still-controversial topic of hormone replacement is so revolutionary you probably have not heard of it before—and quite possibly your busy primary care physician hasn't either.

With awareness comes opportunity for new action. This means you have to take the lead. If you want the next twenty, thirty, or forty years of life to be a *hell of a lot* better than your first twenty, thirty, or forty years of life, you must assume personal responsibility for understanding your options and making informed decisions. Begin right now to make choices that will recalibrate your chronological age and override any hardwired, negative genetic coding. Again, I am here to help.

For the last five years I have worked with Randy to refine a holistic approach to turning back your inner clock at a cellular level. We begin with a methodology for determining the age of your ovaries, or how much older you are without them, then provide a four-step plan to recover years while also decelerating ongoing aging. Our four steps are:

1. Our Belly Flat Diet—including foods and supplements—nutritionally engineered to eliminate age- and hormone-related belly fat and keep it off for good;
2. A fun exercise strategy to decrease the overabundance of estrogen and to counter fat-packing stress hormones;
3. A strategy for eliminating toxins in your home that dangerously mimic estrogen;
4. And, when lifestyle choices alone are not enough, a natural, medically supervised approach to restoring needed hormone levels eroded by age and stress.

If you stick to this plan indefinitely, you will feel and look better as the years roll by. It will improve your health, flatten your tummy, give your face a more youthful glow, and increase your zest for what's yet to come. Is there any reason you should not get started today?

CHAPTER 1

HOW OLD ARE YOUR OVARIES (OR HOW MUCH OLDER ARE YOU WITHOUT THEM)?

WHEN THE SECOND EDITION our book, *From Hormone Hell to Hormone Well,* was awarded the 2010 Bronze National Consumer Health Information Award, I was instantly a speaker in demand. At one private girls' high school alumnae luncheon, the audience nodded, laughed, passed tissues, took notes, and gave me a standing ovation. I was preparing to head to the airport when Hannah, dean of students, asked if I had a few minutes. The door to her office barely shut before she broke down.

"I'm only forty-two but I feel—and know I look—much older. I've been dean for seven years, every year setting an enrollment record. Early on I secured the opportunity for our school to participate in a national study examining the benefits and pitfalls of learning in a single-gender environment. Released in 2009, the results put this school on the map.

"The study showed girls graduating from single-gender schools expressed more confidence in their math, computer, writing, and communication skills than girls attending independent coeducational high schools. Overnight we shifted from being a well-respected local girls' school to one of the most sought-after educational destinations for young women across the United States.

"Now should be the high point of my career. Instead, I feel stale, and my performance is lethargic. At home, I'm short-tempered and unenthused. My mother was a gifted pediatrician, but once she turned forty, she got fat and depressed, eventually losing all steam about her life's purpose. Is that my future?"

Many women share this woman's fears. Your mother's experience does not have to dictate yours. Hormones are no slam-dunk anecdote for what you are going through, but based on medical science and clinical evidence, a combination of lifestyle choices and natural hormone replacement will likely be a critical variable in turning you around.

HOW OUR OVARIES AGE

Chronological age is not necessarily the age of our ovaries. This is an important differentiation because ovaries are the chief production plant for our sex hormones, that is, estrogen, testosterone, and progesterone. The "older" our ovaries are, the fewer sex hormones they can produce and the more rapidly we age.

Clinical studies evidence how hormones are chemical messengers needed for life. At different ages and life cycles, hormones foster puberty, contribute to fertility, and support reproductive health.

While less well understood within the traditional medical community, breakthrough clinical research out of such respected medical schools as Harvard and Emory University prove that optimum hormone balance should be considered a critical variable in a lifetime strategy for breast, heart, bone, and brain health.

Insufficient hormone levels do more than trigger the onset of menopause. When hormone levels begin to wane and sputter as early as a woman's thirties, the negative impact is physical, mental, and emotional. Ovaries age more rapidly, and therein begin to slow down hormone production earlier, if you had:

- Your first menstrual cycle before age twelve,
- Your first child in your late teens or twenties,
- Multiple children,
- Long-term exposure to xenohormones, for example, synthetic, biochemically foreign hormones commonly found in our environment.

Aging accelerates even more when your aging body's lagging hormone levels shift you into natural menopause, or if you experience the shock of sudden menopause after a partial or complete hysterectomy.

HOW MANY DAMN "PAUSES" ARE THERE?

Thirty-six-year-old Lily sat down in Randy's office. "I feel as if I am having an out-of-body experience. I snap at the kids, don't give a crap about work, and daydream about dark chocolate bars with sea salt rather than when my husband and I can have an evening alone. My oldest sister suggested I get my hormones checked, but she is fifty-two and through menopause. My periods are still regular, but a girlfriend said I might be premenopausal or perimenopausal. Just how many damn 'pauses' are there?"

After scrutinizing Lily's lab results, Randy revealed that her hormone profile and symptoms validated that she had moved from her "reproductive years" to a cycle medically termed "premenopause." Many women and their doctors misdiagnose this life cycle because periods remain regular. In five to ten years, a shift in Lily's hormone level profile, along with irregular menstrual cycles, will shift her from "premenopause" into "perimenopause."

Whether you are a regularly menstruating, slightly pudgier, more irritable, low-libido-suffering *premenopausal gal;* a hot flashing, night sweating, irregular bleeding *perimenopausal lady;* an increasingly depressed *menopausal woman* experiencing loss of bone density, painful vaginal dryness, and increased risk of heart disease; or a *postmenopausal matriarch* doing crossword puzzles to ward off dementia, it is essential you understand how cellular-level shifts in hormone balance dictate your health and well-being.

As women, we physically, biochemically, mentally, and sexually peak in our twenties, plateau in our thirties, and begin a sharp descent in our forties. Recall, between age forty and fifty is "the decade of vulnerability." Age fifty and beyond, the harder we have to work to reverse negative trends already in motion. Now let's examine the role our hormones—or lack of them—play.

In the Age of Arrogance, our twenties, hormone production is typically jamming, meaning levels of all sex hormones—estrogen, progesterone, and testosterone—are optimum. You start the negative aging trend when, as you move into your thirties, your ovaries are unable to produce as many needed hormones as they once could.

Age of Reality thirty-something women are particularly at risk for a medical condition termed "estrogen dominance." Because progesterone levels are the first to slow down, declining 120 times more rapidly than estrogen levels, the ovaries are producing way more estrogen than can be balanced by diminished progesterone levels. Common symptoms of estrogen dominance in the thirty-something woman include worsened premenstrual syndrome (PMS); weight gain around the belly, butt, hips, and thighs; decreased energy, loss of sex drive, and onset of headaches or migraines around the period. Clinical studies show lack of progesterone also negatively impacts breast, heart, bone, and brain health.

Premenopausal women in their thirties and early forties having regular periods are most likely to be misdiagnosed. Rather than recognize the symptoms, test hormone levels, and treat hormone imbalances accordingly, many medical professionals miss the boat. Instead they Band-Aid the underlying issue with a prescription for an antidepressant or diet pill. In the United States, ob-gyns—not mental health professionals—are the number-one prescriber of antidepressants.

During the Age of Vulnerability, the forties, hormones act in a stop-go, up-down hormone popcorn popper. Women in their forties having irregular periods are perimenopausal, literally meaning "around menopause." During these years, progesterone levels decline even more significantly while estrogen levels become sporadic, sometimes high peaks, other times low troughs. Without stable estrogen, menstruation doesn't occur regularly and vaginal tissue can atrophy (weaken), making lubrication difficult and intercourse painful.

Testosterone levels also begin to decline in our "decade of vulnerability." When testosterone production sputters, usually mid- to late forties, women suffer loss of energy, decreased sex drive, loss of muscle tone, and less experience of sexual pleasure.

Fifty-one, the official launch of our "Now or Never" years, is the average age women in the United States enter menopause. Clinically, menopause is defined as not having had a period for a year or more. Our aging ovaries may still sporadically sputter, but levels of all three sex hormones—estrogen, progesterone, and testosterone—are in the toilet. We do not look or feel as good as we once did. Skin becomes dry and wrinkly; vaginas do not lubricate easily. Worse, health risks increase. Ongoing/untreated hormone-level decline is clinically linked with an increased risk of breast and endometrial cancers, heart attack, stroke, osteoporosis, and Alzheimer's disease.

Do nothing to boost lagging hormone levels and you stack the cards for a fatter, more disease-prone, emotionally labile, increasingly sexless, and potentially senile future.

LIKE MOTHER, LIKE DAUGHTER
. . . OR NOT?

Like Hannah, I spent years worrying my menopause would mimic my mother's. Mother was the baby in a family of five children. Her daddy, Franklin Kingsley Sandusky, ran mills, first in Alabama and later Florida, that manufactured the tops of wooden barrels. At some point there was an accident. The fingers of his right hand were cut off on the assembly line. He was soon out of work. Granddaddy Sandusky then took up farming outside a little hiccup town called Bonifay, Florida. There was not much money. As a teenager, my mother was a hot one to handle, smoking cigarettes at school and sneaking out of her bedroom window at night.

Mother wanted to go to college but they couldn't afford it. She got a scholarship to a secretarial training program and lined up a waitress job to cover expenses. Sadly, Granddaddy Sandusky wouldn't allow it. I'm told Grandmother Sandusky didn't have much say. At nineteen, Betty Frank married her high-school sweetheart, June Terry.

At twenty, Betty Frank Terry gave birth to a six-pound gumdrop named Sheila. At twenty-four, she learned June had testicular cancer. At twenty-five she was a widow . . . with a five-year-old and a $110-per-month life insurance check.

Now what? Not much money, no education or skills, living in a town without a stoplight. What were her options?

You guessed right. At twenty-seven, my mother wed my father, Angus Douglas Williams, Jr., becoming Betty Frank Williams. Four years later, I was born.

For the next ten years, we were a happy family. We moved to Panama City, Florida, where Daddy worked as an Allstate Insurance salesman. I was severely asthmatic in my early childhood, and my pediatrician advised Mother that I shouldn't play any running games or sports. I was so overprotected, I had few playmates but entertained myself with a menagerie of pets—including a chicken named Bambam and a skunk named Violet—in our backyard.

Sometime in her early forties, something inside Mother soured. She began complaining of bruising headaches and had frequent, extreme mood swings and violent outbursts. After some of the worst, she seemed dazed and perplexed by the havoc in her wake. I've since learned, sadly from personal experience, that something of an amnesic fugue can occur with severe migraines.

To the outside world, we continued to be that "happy family" involved in the community and attending church. Yet from about ten years old until I escaped to college at seventeen, my life was a terror-breathing house of mirrors. Some days Mother was my most loving advocate, instructor of beauty, and strategic life coach. Too often, however, she was an irrational, raging shrew . . . a woman of whom I was afraid.

In Mother's early fifties, she calmed down and came back to herself, as if an exorcism had occurred. At first shyly, then diligently, she made peace with the women she loved most: Sheila, me, and her sister. There were emotional scars, but over time and with love we rediscovered faith in family and the magic of memory-making. Mother and I even went on a three-week girl-trip cruise to Greece. Then Mother, at only sixty-four, had a sudden heart attack and died.

Today I fully believe my mother was literally a victim, a marionette, of her hormones—or lack thereof. It is also clinically probable that an underlying hormone imbalance contributed to her heart disease. All evidence points to her suffering an extreme hormone disorder at a cellular level that jettisoned with the onset of perimenopause. The fact that her extreme behavior abated after menopause supports this premise.

I am determined that my life will be calmer and longer and have a happier ending. Mother's story is my motivation to understand all I can about how hormone levels shift with age and what can be done to turn that around. The next chapters share with you what I know now.

CHAPTER 2

Step 1: Get Rid of Belly Fat for Good

Your belly fat is aging you right now. It is also increasing your risk of developing a chronic disease. If you are overweight, advice to "eat less and exercise more" probably makes you want to either cry or spit. Sadly, if you are older than thirty-five, you are likely in this crowd. Medical statistics show that women will gain an average of one to two pounds every year from the age of thirty-five to fifty-five.

> Women will gain an average of one to two pounds every year from the age of thirty-five to fifty-five.

Consider both Wendy's and Almeda's frustration: Forty-three-year-old Wendy sobbed in the shower. Tonight she and Saj were attending an Athena Awards ceremony where Saj's mother Almeda was an honoree, but despite starving herself for weeks, Wendy still couldn't zip up a single pre-baby outfit. If she wore a maternity dress, people were bound to ask, "When are you due?" She would feel the fool telling them, "My baby's two years old."

A few miles away, sixty-one-year-old Almeda stepped into her evening-out uniform, a plus-size 18 Eileen Fisher black pantsuit. She looked in the mirror, sighed, and reached for a brightly colored shawl. *Maybe this shawl will hide my rolls of back fat. A few more years of unstoppable weight gain and I'll be buying clothes from a custom tent store.*

Wendy and Almeda are not alone. A study funded by the Centers for Disease Control (CDC) and released May 2012 indicates that more than 30 percent of American adults are now overweight and 34 percent are obese. By 2030, a projected 42 percent of American adults will be obese and 11 percent will be severely obese.

What is the link between getting older and fatter? More critically, is there anything to be done to reverse this trend? Our medically proven premise is this: Those extra pounds creeping up and cementing around your middle have little to do with your inability to diet properly, limit carbs, walk an extra mile, or do more crunches; they have everything to do with an age-related shift in hormone production. And, *yes*, this book can help you turn that around.

HORMONE IMBALANCE SABOTAGES YOUR WAISTLINE

Odds are you were most fit and svelte in your twenties. Your "reproductive years" is the season of life when your hormones are in optimum balance, biologically stimulating you to procreate and conceive. The mix of essential hormones includes the sex hormones (estrogen, progesterone, and testosterone), as well as FSH (folli-cle-stimulating hormone), LH (luteinizing hormone), and GnRH (gonadotropin-releasing hormone). These interact as if in an intri-cate symphony, each playing a unique yet interdependent function within your body and brain.

Within the ovaries are follicles that store eggs, or ova. In her early twenties, a woman has approximately four hundred thousand folli-cles. By the mid-thirties, the number of follicles has fallen from four hundred thousand follicles to approximately twenty-five thousand. Each follicle releases another chemical messenger, Inhibin B, whose function is to literally "inhibit" the ovaries' production of estro-gen. The fewer follicles, the less Inhibin B in your system, the more estrogen produced by the ovaries, sometimes up to 30 percent more than what was produced by the ovaries in the reproductive years. Simultaneously, progesterone production begins to decline at a rate 120 times faster than estrogen levels. As described in Chapter 1, this imbalance between rising estrogen and declining progesterone levels is clinically termed "estrogen dominance."

Estrogen dominance fosters weight gain around the belly, butt, hips, and thighs, and then—double whammy—body fat produces even more estrogen.

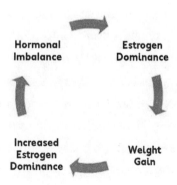

Hormonal Imbalance → Estrogen Dominance → Weight Gain → Increased Estrogen Dominance →

This cycle continues throughout the thirties, forties, fifties, and beyond. Even during and after menopause, estrogen dominance is still a concern.

Many women make the mistake of thinking that if they are no longer having regular menstrual cycles, they no longer have to worry about sabotaging hormone levels or the lack thereof. This is wrong. It is a misconception to believe that once you stop having periods, your ovaries turn off like a light switch.

Although menopause indicates a drastic shift in your body's hormonal equilibrium, it does not mean that your sex hormones have completely evaporated from your body. The ovaries of a menopausal woman are still quite active, producing 40 to 60 percent of the estrogen produced in younger years. Progesterone and testosterone production, however, will continue to decline.

If you are a woman who has entered an abrupt, artificial menopause as a result of a complete or partial hysterectomy, you can still be estrogen dominant. Even though you no longer have ovaries, your body fat is still producing estrogen.

As your body's progesterone production decreases with age and estrogen becomes dominant, your body releases insulin more rapidly and more often. Insulin is the hormone within your body primarily responsible for metabolism and fat storage. Most of the actions of insulin are directed at metabolism (control) of carbohydrates (sugars and starches), lipids (fats), and proteins. When fluctuating hormones unnaturally stimulate insulin release, you get hungry faster and often crave sugar. In fact, insulin-triggered food cravings can sometimes be uncontrollable, causing you to ingest more calories and pack on even more pounds.

ESTROGEN DOMINANCE TIES
UP TESTOSTERONE

Age-related hormonal discordance gets worse for your waist-line. Estrogen levels that are too high stimulate an increase of sex hormone binding globulin (SHBG) two to three times the normal levels. SHBG then circulates through your bloodstream, tying up free testosterone like Velcro, therein negatively impacting healthy weight and body mass composition. Sexual desire and experience of pleasure also decrease. In your late forties and early fifties, the ovaries further decline in testosterone production, predisposing you to an even bigger, bulging middle.

ESTROGEN DOMINANCE DISRUPTS
THYROID FUNCTION

The thyroid gland is best known for its metabolic function, which affects weight. Statistics show that one in eight women between the ages of thirty-five and sixty-five, and one in five women older than sixty-five, have some form of thyroid disease. Hyperthyroidism results from the body producing too much thyroid hormone, but far more common is hypothyroidism, the result of not making enough thyroid hormone. Of similar impact at a cellular level, estrogen dominance renders the thyroid dysfunctional, causing your body's metabolism to slow down. The resulting condition is called *relative hypothyroidism*.

Undetected and untreated, thyroid disorders can not only cause weight gain, they can lead to heart disease, osteoporosis, and other serious health problems. About 26 percent of women in their mid- to late forties are diagnosed with some type of thyroid condition. Younger women are also at risk. Ten percent of women will have thyroid dysfunction following pregnancy. New mothers often ignore their symptoms, attributing them to postpartum depression—just as middle-age women attribute their symptoms to menopause. Consider thirty-two-year-old Cassie and fifty-one-year-old Ruth: six months after Olivia was born, Cassie continued to feel low, not like herself. Looking in the mirror made it worse. Her once-shapely form remained in a pudgy caterpillar shape. She cried continuously but snapped Duane's head off when he asked how he could help. Not sure what to do, Duane called his mother to come.

Instead of helping Cassie with the baby, however, Ruth ran between unfinished projects and the bathroom, where she constantly filled diaper pails with blood-soaked maxipads. She was so irritable that Cassie kept Olivia in a portable crib in her bedroom and only came out to fight with Ruth over the thermostat.

Duane confided to his best friend, "The baby is great, but when it comes to Mom and Cassie, I don't know whether to call a doctor, personal trainer, or a shrink."

Bottom line: age-related hormone imbalance, particularly estrogen dominance, is fueling the elastic jeans industry. Five pounds can quickly morph to twenty, thirty, or more. If this is happening to you, you've got bigger issues than elastic versus zippers. Your health is in jeopardy.

ESTROGEN DOMINANCE IS A HEALTH RISK

The trouble with estrogen-related belly fat is that it not only makes you unhappy with how you look, it makes you feel lousy, puts your health at risk, and accelerates your aging. Estrogen-related belly fat is not limited to the extra layer of padding located just below the skin (subcutaneous fat). It also includes visceral fat, which lies deep inside your abdomen, surrounding your internal organs. Although subcutaneous fat poses cosmetic concerns, visceral fat is associated with far more dangerous health consequences. This is because an excessive amount of visceral fat produces hormones and other substances that can raise blood pressure, negatively alter good and bad cholesterol levels, and impair the body's ability to use insulin (insulin resistance). All of this can increase the risk of serious health problems, including:

- Breast cancer
- Cardiovascular disease
- Stroke
- Type 2 diabetes
- Colorectal cancer

Recent research also shows that women in their forties who have belly fat are more likely to get Alzheimer's and other forms of dementia in their seventies. Other studies link belly fat to an increased risk of premature death—regardless of overall weight.

Speaking of Aging Too Fast . . . Estrogen Dominance and Precocious Puberty

About 1 in 5,000 children experience early puberty. Studies suggest that, on average, kids are starting puberty earlier than they once did. Could the rise in obesity be playing a role? Many experts think so, at least when it comes to girls.

"I think it's quite clear that some of the early puberty we're see-ing is related to obesity," says Paul Kaplowitz, MD, PhD, chief of the division of endocrinology at Children's National Medical Center in Washington, DC. "It's not the whole story, but it's a factor."

The excess fatty tissue produces higher estrogen levels, which leads to greater insulin resistance, causes girls to have more body fat, and then produces more estrogen. Just as with older women, the estrogen-belly-fat-estrogen cycle feeds on itself, speeding up aging for preadolescent girls.

BELLY FLAT DIET ELIMINATES ESTROGEN DOMINANCE

Over the last decade, I have worked with Randy to hone in on the link between an underlying condition of estrogen dominance and age-related belly fat to offer women a solution. Our Belly Flat Plan begins with our Belly Flat Diet. Our clinically vetted, nutri-tional approach is biochemically engineered to eliminate the fat-generating extra estrogen in your system.

Our Belly Flat Diet is a unique version of the Mediterranean way of eating, with extra emphasis on foods proven to decrease your extra estrogen load. The traditional Mediterranean diet empha-sizes healthy fats from nuts, fish, and vegetable oils; fruits, veggies, whole grains, beans, nuts, legumes, olive oil, and flavorful herbs and spices; eating fish and seafood at least a couple of times a week; enjoying poultry, eggs, cheese, and yogurt in moderation; and sav-ing sweets and red meat for special occasions. Like Randy, most doctors agree it is fine to top off with a splash wine in moderation (if you want).

We recommend adding to the Mediterranean diet specific "belly-blaster" foods proven to melt away unwanted pounds and inches. Follow our diet and you can lose those extra pounds around your middle once and for all. If you are in your thirties and just beginning to worry about a muffin top or love handles, our Belly Flat Diet can put your fears to rest for life.

Your smaller waist will be one very noticeable benefit. Another less obvious but very real bonus of losing those pounds once and forever will be decreasing your risk of the previously named chronic diseases and very likely extending your life span.

DAILY BELLY BLASTER FOODS

Cruciferous Vegetables and Indole-3-Carbinol (I3C)

Eating a variety of cruciferous vegetables is key to losing and keeping off belly fat. How estrogen is metabolized in the body is determined by an individual's biochemical makeup, with some people producing more 2-hydroxy derivatives (the "good" estrogens) and others producing more 4- and 16-hydroxyesterone (the "bad" estrogens). Consuming large amounts of cruciferous vegetables, such as broccoli, asparagus, cauliflower, spinach, Brussels sprouts, celery, beet root, kale, cabbage, parsley root, radish, turnip, and collard and mustard greens, has been shown to improve the production of "good" estrogen and foster an optimum 2/16 estrogen ratio.

Biochemically, here's what happens: cruciferous vegetables contain a phytonutrient called indole-3-carbinol (I3C). I3C has been shown to act as a catalyst to pull estrone down a benign pathway to 2-hydroxy estrone, thus decreasing levels of the carcinogenic 4- and 16-alpha-hydroxyestrone. To put it simply, this means that cruciferous vegetables can help decrease the body's load of unhealthy estrogens and reduce an overall unhealthy condition of estrogen dominance.

Citrus Fruits: D-Limonene

D-limonene, found in the oils of citrus fruits, has been shown to promote detoxification of estrogen. Common citrus fruits include oranges, grapefruit, tangerines, lemons, limes, and tangelos. Research also found that, when administered an extract of D-limonene, both male and female lab mice evidenced lower body weight.

Insoluble Fiber

There are two types of fiber: soluble and insoluble. Soluble fiber dissolves in water and is degraded by bacteria in your colon. It forms a gel in your intestines, which regulates the flow of waste material through your digestive tract. This type of fiber is found in oatmeal, oat bran, dried peas, beans, lentils, apples, pears, strawberries, and blueberries. Soluble fiber is good for you, but no matter how much of it you eat, it won't influence your hormonal equilibrium.

Insoluble fiber, on the other hand, can directly impact your hormone balance by helping decrease estrogen overload. Insoluble fiber binds to extra estrogen in the digestive tract. This extra estrogen is later eliminated in the body through the feces. According to the Harvard School of Public Health, sources of insoluble fiber include whole grains, whole-wheat breads, barley, couscous, brown rice, whole-grain breakfast cereals, wheat bran, seeds, carrots, cucumbers, zucchini, celery, and tomatoes.

Lignans

Ground or milled flaxseed, sesame seeds, and flaxseed oil are part of a food group called lignans. The friendly bacteria in our intestines convert plant lignans into the "human" lignans, primarily enterolactone, that have a weak estrogenlike activity. When there are low estrogen levels in the body, these weak lignan "estrogens" make up some of the insufficiency. When the body is estrogen dominant, however, the lignan "estrogens" bind to the human body's estrogen receptors, thereby reducing human estrogen activity at a cellular level.

Oily Fish

Fish oil, rich in omega-3 fatty acids, assists with the production of many hormones. Oily fish, such as salmon, sardines, and herring, all have high levels of omega-3 fatty acids, which have been shown to have a weak estrogenic effect. Cellular binding of omega-3 fatty acids "tricks" the body into reducing an underlying condition of estrogen dominance.

The role of omega-3 fatty acids is of particular note in the production of testosterone. According to a 2011 study published in the *American Journal of Clinical Nutrition*, eating a diet rich in oily fish can improve body-fat ratio by promoting muscle protein synthesis.

You will find tasty recipes in Appendix A. Follow our Belly Flat Diet Plan for just four weeks for a tighter tummy, rebalanced body, and recharged life.

Blast Away Your Belly Fat: Foods that Reduce Your Extra Estrogen Load

Cruciferous Vegetables: Eat 2 to 3 servings a day (broccoli, asparagus, cauliflower, spinach, Brussels sprouts, celery, alfalfa, beet root, kale, cabbage, parsley root, radish, turnip, collard and mustard greens)

Citrus Fruits: Eat 1 serving a day (oranges, grapefruit, tangerines, lemons, limes, and tangelos)

Insoluble Fiber: Eat 2 servings a day (whole grains, whole wheat breads, barley, couscous, brown rice, whole-grain breakfast cereals, wheat bran, seeds, carrots, cucumbers, zucchini, celery, and tomatoes)

Lignans: Eat 2 to 3 tablespoons a day (ground or milled flaxseed, sesame seeds, or flaxseed oil)

Oily Fish: Eat 2 to 3 servings per week (salmon, herring, mackerel, and sardines)

CHAPTER 3

STEP 2:
MOVE AND GROOVE

S TEP 2 OF THE BELLY FLAT PLAN requires you to get up and get moving. While you are likely well aware of how exercise burns calories, you may be startled to review the science proving how regular, strenuous exercise helps reduce estrogen dominance, decrease health-risky stress hormones, and decelerate aging at a DNA level.

EXERCISE DECREASES
ESTROGEN DOMINANCE

In 2007, the Penn Ovarian Aging Study showed that the more women exercised, the healthier their estrogen-progesterone ratio. Studies in such respected medical publications as the *Journal of the National Cancer Institute* and *Cancer Epidemiology Biomarkers Preview* have shown that after twelve months of regular exercise (thirty minutes/five days per week), unhealthy estrogen levels drop an average of 13 percent.

In another 2010 study, postmenopausal women who regularly did intense exercise for a year had lower levels of estrogen compared to women who didn't exercise. Before joining the study, most of the 320 postmenopausal women ages fifty to seventy-four were overweight and did very little or no exercise. The women were randomly split into two groups: half the women kept up their usual level of activity during the one-year study; half the women did intense aerobic exercise for about 225 minutes (4 hours and 45 minutes) each week during the study.

The women in the exercise group usually worked out for about forty-five minutes three to five days per week. At least three sessions each week were done with trainers at a fitness center and the rest of the exercise was done at home. The exercise was intense and raised the women's heart rates to a target level above resting heart rate.

The researchers measured the women's levels of several hormones and a related protein at the beginning of the study, in the middle of the study (six months), and at the end of the study (one year). At the end of one year, the levels of estrogen were 7 to 9 percent lower in the women in the exercise program compared to the women who kept up their usual slack activity level.

EXERCISE COUNTERS
FAT-PACKING STRESS HORMONES

Stress can make you tense and sick. It can also make you fat. Exercise counters all three.

Your adrenal glands produce three stress hormones: adrenaline, cortisol, and DHEA. Short-term, urgent stress—such as seeing your five-year-old reach for a hot skillet or having your husband ask you to watch him skydive—triggers a rush of adrenaline. Long-term, chronic stress has a different impact at a cellular level.

Chronic stress is defined as a circumstance that exists for three months or more. Some more common chronic stressors for women include ongoing financial pressures, single motherhood, caring for an ill and aging parent, attempting to juggle a heavy workload and home life, or attempting to discipline an irascible teenager. Chronic stress causes the adrenal glands to first produce an overabundance of cortisol, then, once this supply is exhausted, cortisol levels plummet. Too high or too low cortisol levels pack even more pounds around your waist.

Numerous studies in the last several decades have confirmed that regular physical activity relieves feelings of stress and, at a cellular level, regulates cortisol production. Being active on a regular basis helps eliminate the threat that surging cortisol levels will contribute to an ever-expanding waistline.

EXERCISE RELEASES FAT-BURNING HORMONE

A hormone released by the muscles during exercise transforms white cells into brown cells, according to research findings published in the June 2012 *Harvard Health Letter*. The hormone, known as irisin, also appears to overcome insulin resistance, a condition leading to type 2 diabetes. White cells simply store fat. Brown cells, in contrast, actually burn fat. And brown cells keep burning fat even after you have stopped exercising.

"Irisin travels throughout the body in the blood and alters fat cells," explains Dr. Anthony Komaroff, editor of the *Harvard Health Letter*. "If your goal is to lose weight and keep it off, you want to exercise with the objective to increase the number of brown fat-burning cells and decrease the number of white fat-storing cells."

Exercise Turns Back Your Cellular Clock

In heartening research published in 2011 in the *Proceedings of the National Academy of Sciences*, exercise reduced or eliminated almost every detrimental effect of aging in mice. The study followed a group of mice from birth. By the time they reached eight months, or their early sixties in human terms, the animals were extremely frail and decrepit, with spindly muscles, shrunken brains, enlarged hearts, shriveled gonads, and patchy, graying fur. Listless, they barely moved around their cages. All were dead before reaching a year of age—except the mice that exercised.

Half of the mice were allowed to run on a wheel for forty-five minutes three times a week, beginning at three months. These rodent runners were required to maintain a fairly brisk pace, the equivalent of a person running a fifty- or fifty-five minute 10K (a 10K race is 6.2 miles). The mice continued this regimen for five months.

At eight months, when their sedentary lab mates were bald, frail, and dying, the running rats remained youthful. They had full pelts of dark fur, no salt-and-pepper shadings. They also had maintained almost all of their muscle mass and brain volume. Their genitalia had not shriveled, and their hearts were as good as new.

Enough about rodents . . . what about women? What does new science say about exercise and aging? A study published in the

January 2008 issue of *Archives of Internal Medicine* confirmed the beneficial impact of exercise at the cellular level. The London-based study was founded on the observation that telomeres (regions of repetitive DNA at the end of a chromosome) in white blood cells erode and shorten during the aging process. Thus, their length and quality are biological indicators of human aging, sort of an internal lifeline. Researchers compared the length and quality of the telomeres in 1,200 sets of twins; within each set, one twin exercised regularly and the other was sedentary.

Researchers found that the longer, healthier telomeres of the active twin indicated a younger biological age—sometimes by as much as nine years—when compared to the biological age indicated by the shorter, degraded telomeres of the sedentary twin.

SIX TIPS TO MOVE MORE

Do a Rooski

Elaine's morning routine of ten minutes of yoga followed by a brisk four-mile walk had kept her trim for twenty-plus years, but between forty-seven and fifty-four, her waist ballooned from size 8 to size 12. She tried leaving jam off her toast, forgoing afternoon cheese and cracker snacks, and walking an extra mile every day—all to no avail. Her dejection was palpable.

"Please tell me there is something else I can do. I can't stand the idea of being stuck with this swollen body for the rest of my life."

Metabolism slows down by 5 percent each decade. Women also lose 6 to 8 percent of muscle mass per decade. This is bad news because muscle burns the most calories. The final kicker: If, like Elaine, you always have the same workout routine, your muscles will adapt. This means that over time your favorite exercise routine will burn fewer and fewer calories.

My approach to outsmarting my muscles is rooski play. "Rooski" is a football term meaning "trick" play. By constantly switching up exercise routines with a variety of new muscle-building, strength-training, and heart-pumping activities, you can keep your muscles constantly guessing—and those calories consistently churning and burning. Sure, you can continue to walk and run, but with options like water aerobics, Zumba dancing, hot yoga, paddleboarding, and rollerblading, there is even more fun to be had.

Buddy Up

Let's face it. Exercising can be boring. Add a friend, spouse, part-ner, or lover to the mix and suddenly being on the treadmill becomes a lot more interesting. Working out together is not only a great way to catch up, but it makes your calorie-burning time go by a lot faster. Whether you're trying out a kickboxing class, running on the track, or logging time on the elliptical trainer, doing it next to a friend means you have someone to talk and laugh with while you sweat.

Take Up a New Sport

In grammar school, no one ever picked me for their kickball team, and my college tennis instructor told me I would be better off playing board games. At fifty-three, could there still be hope that I might find a sport that motivated me more toward fitness? Consider these role models: Academy Award–winning actress Geena Davis has stated that she was not an athlete growing up and that her introduction to archery was in 1997. Two years later, Davis was one of three hundred women who vied for a semifinals berth in the US Olympic archery team to participate in the Sydney 2000 Summer Olympics. Don't think of archery as stationary. While it may not be an aerobic sport, it is a great workout for shoulders, back, and abdominal core muscles.

Kathy Martin, a busy working mother who had never competed at a track meet, started running in her late forties. In September 2011, she turned sixty. In the year that followed, Kathy ran in thirteen highly competitive races, including the Chicago Marathon and a cross-country championship in Seattle, and she set nine American and two world records.

In 2012, ninety-three-year-old Tao Porchon-Lynch was awarded the Guinness Book of World Records title of world's oldest yoga instructor. Tao's been teaching yoga for sixty-one years, and it has kept her in amazing shape. She loves doing it, saying, "I am going to teach yoga until I can't breathe anymore. Then it's going to carry me to the next planet. I love yoga. It brightens my day, and it makes everybody smile." Even after having a hip replacement, Tao's still more nimble than many of her students. Oh, if you think yoga is not a "team sport," Tao has more to offer. She's also a competitive dancer in tango competitions and partners with a man who is a whopping sixty-nine years younger.

Post Goals for Friends and Followers

Telling your mirror about your exercise plan may not keep you as focused as posting the proclamation to all 248 of your Facebook friends or tweeting it to dozens of followers. For New Jersey resident Colleen Lange, forty-one, what started out as a little weight-loss contest between a few close friends on Facebook grew into a group of more than twenty participants from four states—some of whom she's never met. "We post daily—sharing recipes, supporting one another, even talking a little smack for extra motivation," she says.

"Connecting with people who share the same goals is like having your very own cheering section," says Rachel Meltzer Warren, RD, a New York–based nutritionist. "There's always someone there to celebrate when you drop those first ten pounds or help you get back on track if you regain three." Personal stories show it works, and the scientific community is paying attention: government-funded studies are under way looking at how technologies like social networking can help young adults achieve healthy weights.

Stay in Your PJs

When I used time as an excuse, my cardiologist, Pam Rama, MD, said, "Work out in your pajamas. Forgo the time and trip to the gym by plugging in a DVD or checking out the On-Demand channel on your television to access a variety of fun, fit exercises. I do it all the time."

While you are in your pjs, consider . . .

Sexercise

Sex burns calories and can fuel weight loss. The average lovemaking session burns between 50 and 100 calories. Having sex three times a week burns 7,500 calories per year. That's the equivalent of jogging seventy-five miles. The more intense the sex, the more calories burned: up to 15,000 calories annually, which equals more than four pounds of fat burned away. In addition, certain sexual positions will strengthen your core, increase flexibility, and tone tummy, tush, and thighs. For details on a few frisky bedroom moves, check out Chapter 9.

CHAPTER 4

STEP 3:
DETOX YOUR HOME

D ISTURBING STUDIES SHOW THAT everyday toxins in your home can disrupt hormone balance, accelerate your aging, and make you and your family sick. Exposure to environmental toxins, called xenohormones, is also emerging as a possible contributor to our fat epidemic.

HOW TOXINS MAKE YOU FAT

The body accumulates weight-inducing toxins from air and water pollution, toxic foods, medications, and many other elements with which we come into contact. When toxins accumulate in the body, the liver and other organ systems try to filter them out of the body as rapidly as they come in. When the liver is overloaded, the body resorts to using fat to insulate the toxins from damaging the body's tissues.

When a person tries to lose weight, it becomes difficult to remove fat that the body is using to protect itself. If a person does find a way to lose the weight, they often will see it come back more quickly, as the body will immediately try to conserve more fat where it was lost. Those who consume the most toxic foods, take medications, and exercise the least will gain weight the fastest.

TOXINS ARE STEALTHY DANGERS

Danika, Randy's daughter and mother of our granddaughter Lulu, called, sounding worried: "I thought breast-feeding Lulu was the best way to get our baby off to a healthy start, but I finished reading this book today. Now I'm scared."

The book, *Breasts: A Natural and Unnatural History*, by Florence Williams, tells the author's story of discovering her own breast milk was loaded with toxins. She says many toxins, including the flame retardants found in her breast milk, leach in from ordinary household items like couches and electronics, which often contain flame retardants. Animal studies have shown certain types of flame retardants interact as xenohormones.

Toxins in Danika's breast milk?

The idea floored me. Nevertheless, I suspected it could be true. While the possibility greatly concerned me, Randy and I encouraged Danika to examine this new information with pragmatism. The short- and long-term health benefits of breast-feeding have long been clinically established. The disturbing reality that xenohormones abound in our everyday environment, potentially accumulating in our bodies and particularly our breasts, should be a call to action. Rather than stop breast-feeding and forgo the proven benefits thereof, a better option could be to determine how women like Danika (and you and me) can decrease exposure to these toxic chemicals on a daily basis.

Hidden Estrogen Mimickers

Persons living in the United States and Western Europe have been found to have much higher estrogen levels than persons living in underdeveloped countries. Environmental estrogen-like hormones in the foods we eat and the chemicals we use are often hidden causative agents of estrogen dominance. Estrogen mimickers in the form of chemicals (xenoestrogens), and foods and plants (phytoestrogens), mimic the action of estrogen produced in cells.

According to Virginia Hopkins, coauthor of Dr. John Lee's *What Your Doctor May Not Tell You About Menopause*, "Most of our exposure to xenohormones comes in very small amounts and any one tiny dose won't have a significant effect. The problem is that most of us are exposed to many tiny doses every day, all day and that has a cumulative effect." The additive effect of years of chronic exposure to environmental estrogens can contribute to a condition of estrogen dominance.

"Xeno" literally means "foreign," therefore xenoestrogens equal foreign estrogens. Xenoestrogens can be found in certain pesticides, herbicides, plastics, fuels, car exhaust, and drugs. Over time, these substances can increase the estrogen load in the body. Xenoestrogens can also be found in many meats and dairy products in the form of chemicals and growth hormones given to the animals.

Some Beauty and Cleaning Products May Harm

Many general hygiene consumer products—such as creams, lotions, soaps, shampoos, perfume, hair spray, and room deodorizers—

contain petrochemicals. These compounds often have chemical structures similar to estrogen and can act like estrogen when introduced into the body. Some shampoos targeted at the African American community even advertise their estrogen content. A 2007 cosmetic industry's chemical safety assessments revealed that 57 percent of baby soaps, 34 percent of body lotions, and 22 percent of all personal care products contained petrochemicals. Need I say more?

Similarly, industrial solvents are another source of xenoestrogens. Industrial solvents are commonly found in cosmetics, fingernail polish, fingernail polish remover, glues, paint, varnishes, cleaning products, carpet, fiberboard, and other processed woods.

Don't Drink the Water

Randy and I reported in *From Hormone Hell to Hormone Well* how just drinking water from a faucet can raise your body's level of xenohormones. According to Marcelle Pick, ob-gyn NP, "Researchers worldwide have observed that fish in our lakes and rivers are actually switching gender due to the high levels of effluent estrogens. Even though mainstream media has only begun to recognize this as 'news,' experts have been discussing the problem of pharmaceutical pollution for more than twenty-five years and have known about 'gender-bent' fish for more than ten years now! Some surmise these changes to be caused in part by excessive levels of steroids—largely excreted by humans using birth control pills and synthetic hormonal replacement therapy (HRT). Our water treatment facilities are not designed to remove hormonal pollutants."

Plastic Disrupts Hormone Balance

Bisphenol A (BPA) is another insidious danger. BPA is a weak synthetic estrogen found in many rigid plastic products, food and formula can linings, dental sealants, and on the shiny side of paper cashier receipts (to stabilize the ink). Its estrogen-like activity makes it a hormone disruptor, like many other chemicals in plastics. Hormone disruptors can affect how estrogen and other hormones act in the body by blocking them or mimicking them, which throws off the body's hormonal balance.

BPA also seems to affect brain development in the womb. In 2011, a study found that pregnant women with high levels of BPA in their urine were more likely to have daughters who showed signs of hyperactivity, anxiety, and depression. The symptoms were seen in girls as young as three.

Limit Consumption of Genetically Modified Organism (GMO) Foods

Most corn and soybean crops grown in the United States are genetically modified, meaning their DNA has been altered to make them more resistant to viruses, bacteria, or insects. GMOs allow farmers to produce larger, healthier crops and make them available at more affordable prices. The uptick in crop production is needed to support rising food demand for a burgeoning populace. The downside is that several studies suggest that GMO foods can have a long-term toxic health impact.

A December 2012 Kaiser Permanente newsletter spoke out against GMOs. The article cautioned that consumers should limit exposure to them by avoiding processed food and, when possible, by choosing organic or "non-GMO" labeled produce.

What Now?

A few years ago Randy and I trademarked Protect the Girls

with the goal of setting forth straightforward steps every woman could do to support her optimum hormone balance, healthy weight, and breast health. Our excellent news is that these same lifestyle actions also support healthy weight and reproductive development for little "girls" in our lives.

- Stick with our Belly Flat Diet for life.
- Exercise more with your daughter(s) and all the little girls you love.
- Buy organic and non-GMO foods when at all possible. Avoid hormone-treated meats and poultry at all costs.
- Drink filtered water. Researchers worldwide have observed fish switching gender due to the high level of effluent estrogen in the water. The problem is attributed to high levels of synthetic hormones excreted by women using synthetic HRT or birth control pills. Our water treatment facilities are not designed to remove hormonal pollutants.
- Drink water from BPA-free containers.
- Never microwave in plastic containers. Avoid using plastic wrap to cover food for microwaving.
- Detox your diet, home, and beauty regimen. "Natural" alternatives can sometimes be pricey. You'll find several terrific resources for money-saving tips for natural and organic living in Appendix B.

CHAPTER 5

STEP 4:
FIND A DOCTOR WHO
CAN HELP

FORTY-NINE-YEAR-OLD ESMERALDA was confused. Over the last ten years her once-fit runner's physique had become mushy around the middle. Revving up for an extra mile and chomping on more celery sticks had no sustainable impact on her midriff flab. Now, constantly miserable with hot flashes and night sweats, she was beginning "The Change." She knew she didn't like how she looked or felt. What she didn't know was what to do about it.

Dr. Ellison, her family's primary care physician for more than two decades, encouraged her to sweat it out but said, "If you must have something, I can write a prescription for a synthetic conjugated estrogen with medroxyprogesterone acetate, but I would want you take it the shortest amount of time possible because of potential side effects."

Lizbeth, her forty-two-year-old sister, thought she had a better answer: "Stay away from those drugs. I just read an article in a magazine while getting my nails done. It said take a supplement called Mexican Wild Yam."

"All bunk," declared best friend Phoebe. "You need to see a doctor who understands and prescribes bioidentical hormones. I've been on them for seven years and have never felt better. But don't take my word for it. Go get your hormone levels tested."

What Our Mothers Couldn't Tell Us and Many Doctors Still Don't Know

No wonder Esmeralda's frustrated. At some point in her life, many women will experience a reality where no matter how committed they are to our Belly Flat Diet, how much they exercise, or how conscientiously they detox their home, unwanted body fat glams back onto the belly and backside, and other uncomfortable symptoms emerge. When this occurs, it means the balance of sex, thyroid, and adrenal hormones has become so off-kilter that lifestyle alone is no longer enough to keep your hormones in balance. It's time for professional medical intervention. If this is your current situation, you must carefully vet the physician or medical professional you choose to help.

For the most part, mainstream medicine continues to view imbalances of life-sustaining hormones as "normal." Most doctors rarely test for hormone levels and blindly reject the idea that restoring hormone profiles to youthful ranges is preventive health and a sound wellness strategy. Years before irregular bleeding, hot flashes, and/or night sweats, symptoms of estrogen dominance can include anxiety, depression, fatigue, headaches (including migraines), worsened premenstrual syndrome (PMS), fuzzy thinking and/or memory loss, breast tenderness, and low libido. As previously described, the consequence of this uninformed viewpoint is that many women are misdiagnosed and prescribed diet pills, diuretics, and/or antidepressants. Others suffer discomforts and diseases largely correctable and preventable.

The reason for the confusion is this: Physicians are not adequately educated in medical school about hormone issues associated with the aging ovary. They have been trained to prescribe synthetic hormone replacement therapy drugs (HRT) that multiple studies in the last ten years have been shown to increase a woman's risk of breast cancer, heart attack, stroke, and dementia. Many physicians are unaware that they have other options to prescribe for their patients.

In the last several years, hormone replacement therapy (HRT) has frequently been in the news, sometimes as the grim reaper of death, other times as the panacea for ageless youth and sexuality. Magazine articles, television shows, and celebrities bandy about terms like "natural," "bioidentical," "synthetic," or "pharmaceutical" as if they were interchangeable. They are not.

"Natural" hormones are those hormones produced within the body by the ovaries, the testes, the adrenal glands, and the hypothalamus. These hormones travel through the bloodstream to fit into specific hormone-receptor sites located throughout the body and brain. Each hormone receptor site will recognize the specific molecular structure of a single type of hormone. This means that a receptor site for progesterone will not recognize estrogen or testosterone; it will only recognize the molecular structure of progesterone.

Hormones produced within your body attach to their receptor sites like keys fitting into locks. The chemical term for this key-and-lock phenomenon is called relative binding affinity (RBA). The hormones your ovaries make have a 100 percent RBA for their respective receptor sites.

WHY BIOIDENTICAL HORMONES ARE SAFE AND SYNTHETIC HORMONES ARE DANGEROUS

Bioidentical hormones are derived from plants (soybeans or wild yams) using biochemistry processes. The biochemical process assures that the molecular structure of bioidentical hormones is identical to that of the natural human hormones once produced by your body. Just like the hormones your ovaries once made, bioidentical hormones have a 100 percent RBA for those hormone-receptor sites throughout your body and brain. When they plug in perfectly, your body and brain once again receive essential chemical messages that only hormones can deliver. Because our bodies recognize, accept, and respond to bioidentical hormones just as they would to hormones from our ovaries, bioidentical hormone replacement therapy (BHRT) is not only safe, it is extremely effective.

It is important to realize that the molecular structure of natural human hormones cannot be patented. Consequently, neither can the identical molecular structure of bioidentical hormones be patented. Without a patent, how could a pharmaceutical company protect its formulation and, most important (to the company), its profits? The answer: They can't. Consequently, for almost three quarters of a century, pharmaceutical companies have been developing, patenting, and marketing hormones that have a slightly different molecular structure from natural human hormones and bioidentical hormones. The pharmaceutically produced and patented hormones should be referred to as synthetic hormones. The list of synthetic hormones on the market today includes such brand names as Premarin, Prempro, Menest, Orthoest, Activella, and Femhrt, among many others.

Synthetic hormones have shapes not seen in nature. Synthetic hormones' poor fit with the body's hormone receptors produces unnatural chemical reactions and striking alterations in biologic activity. As a result, their RBA is less than 100 percent, resulting in side effects and health risks. Premarin, for instance, is metabolized horse estrogen with a low affinity for binding with any human hormone receptor. Premarin is also composed of 49.3 percent of the cancer-promoting estrogen estrone (E1). This is almost ten times the ratio that occurs naturally within the body.

In July 2002, the National Institutes of Health (NIH) halted a large, in-progress study examining the effects of the widely used synthetic hormone replacement therapy medication Prempro, which combines the altered molecular structures for both estrogen and progesterone. (Note: synthetic progesterone is referred to as "progestin.") The study, one of five major studies that made up the large clinical trial called the Women's Health Initiative (WHI), was discontinued because the synthetic hormones were found to increase a woman's risk of breast cancer, as well as heart disease, blood clots, and stroke. Later findings linked synthetic hormone replacement to an increased risk for Alzheimer's disease. Findings were published in the *Journal of the American Medical Association (JAMA)*.

Over the last decade, irrefutable data substantiating the dangers of synthetic hormone replacement has continued to mushroom. The following is excerpted from Prempro's product label warning:

"Using [synthetic, conjugated from horse urine] estrogens with [synthetic] progestins may increase your chance of getting heart attack, stroke, breast cancer or blood clots.

Using [synthetic, conjugated from horse urine] estrogens with [synthetic] progestins may increase your chance of dementia. Using [synthetic, conjugated from horse urine] estrogen alone, e.g., Premarin, may increase your chance of getting cancer of the uterus. What is the most important information I should know about PREMPRO and PREMPHASE (combinations of estrogens and a progestin)?

Do not use estrogens with progestins to prevent heart disease, heart attacks, strokes, or dementia (decline of brain function)

Using estrogens with progestins may increase your chances of getting heart attacks, strokes, breast cancer, or blood clots

Using estrogens with progestins may increase your chance of getting dementia, based on a study of women age 65 years or older

Do not use estrogen alone to prevent heart disease, heart attacks, or dementia

Using estrogen alone may increase your chance of getting cancer of the uterus (womb)

Using estrogen alone may increase your chances of getting strokes or blood clots

Using estrogen alone may increase your chance of getting dementia, based on a study of women age 65 years or older

You and your healthcare provider should talk regularly about whether you still need treatment with PREMPRO or PREMPHASE."

If bioidentical hormone replacement is safe and has been proven to have multiple, positive, long-term health benefits, you may wonder why more physicians continue to recommend and prescribe synthetic hormones versus BHRT. The answer is a mix of ignorance, confusion, and marketing hype.

RANDY'S STORY

Like every other physician of his generation, Randy was trained in medical school to prescribe synthetic hormones, the then-popular Premarin and Prempro, and he did for his first few years after he opened his medical practice. Early on, however, he became greatly concerned by the side effects he observed in his patients, for example, the weight gain, fibrocystic breasts, and increased mood swings. Convinced these could be early road signs for later health disasters, he began to research a safer alternative.

Prior to attending medical school, Randy was a compounding pharmacist specializing in pharmacognosy, that is, natural, plant-based medicines. He drew on this background and also reached out to physician researchers, including Dr. John Lee (author of *What Your Doctor May Not Tell You About Menopause* and *What Your Doctor May Not Tell You About Breast Cancer*) and Dr. Joel Hargrove, then chief of the Department of Reproductive Medicine at Vanderbilt University.

"After reading Dr. Lee's books and reviewing Dr. Hargrove's research, I was fully convinced BHRT was the safest and most efficacious therapeutic option for my patients suffering symptoms of hormone level decline. This was 1996. I was certain that in a year or two, BHRT would be as common a protocol among my physician peers as performing routine pap smears or washing hands before and after a patient's physical exam."

Unfortunately, the traditional medical community was slow to wake up. For more than a decade, Randy's peers ostracized him for prescribing "that bioidentical snake oil." Their unfounded derision cost him more than his pride. In 2003, Randy called me one night from his truck. He was crying. "They said if I don't stop prescribing BHRT, I'm out."

Randy had just left the board meeting of North Florida OB/GYN, a physicians' group-practice-without-walls of which he was a partner. These types of organized physician groups benefit members by centralizing business functions (such as billing, human resources, and payroll), using their combined purchasing strength to negotiate lower costs of medical supplies and negotiating higher reimbursement, for example, payment from insurance companies.

In the 1980s I served as executive vice president for Principal-Care, a company that bought and sold ob-gyn practices, so I was readily familiar with how these organizations work. I understood immediately that if Randy exited this group and went solo, the financial impact would be humongous.

"Randy, this is a big deal. Maybe you should reconsider. If you have to take on responsibilities for all those business functions, I can guarantee your overhead costs are going to increase by a minimum of 30 percent, and how much insurance companies will pay you will decrease by 40. That's a 70 percent negative financial hit."

He did not hesitate.

"My patients matter more than money. Synthetic hormones harm women, put their lives at risk. BHRT is literally life-giving. I don't have a choice. I'll have to figure the business stuff out on my own."

By choosing to continue to prescribe BHRT for his patients despite looming detrimental business and financial implications, Randy stayed true to the spirit of the Hippocratic Oath by not harming his patients.

In 2008–9 two unlikely champions shifted the science of BHRT into the spotlight. Soon, many of those same physicians who had shunned Randy were calling for advice.

TWO UNLIKELY BEDFELLOWS

The about-face in how the traditional medical community diagnoses and treats hormone imbalances has been galvanized by two unlikely bedfellows: respected Republican senator Charles Grassley and revered Democrat Oprah Winfrey.

In December 2008, Senator Grassley wrote pharmaceutical giant Wyeth about the company's practice of medical ghostwriting. The senator then initiated an investigation and obtained documents from recent lawsuits involving Wyeth's synthetic hormone therapy products, for example, the Premarin and Prempro family of drugs, showing how Wyeth hired a medical communications and education company, DesignWrite, to draft review articles regarding the breast cancer risk of hormone therapy. In other words, Wyeth paid DesignWrite to produce legitimate-appearing medical articles saying only those things the company wanted doctors to believe.

Did you just gasp? If you didn't, consider this: because doctors across the United States were fed inaccurate information about the safety of synthetic hormone drugs, millions of women's lives were put at risk—very possibly your own or that of a woman you love.

Senator Grassley had the gonads to take on Big Pharma. He and the US Senate Special Committee on Aging chairman and Wisconsin Democrat Herb Kohl drafted the Physician Payments Sunshine Act, signed into law in 2011. This law now requires public disclosure of all financial relationships between physicians and the pharmaceutical, medical device, and biologics industries, a big step toward pharmaceutical company transparency and truth in advertising.

In 2009, Oprah brought the conversation to a crescendo. "The veil has been lifted," she declared on air, describing her personal experience with BHRT. "If you are planning on living past thirty-five, this is something you need to know."

Oprah interviewed medical expert Christiane Northrup, MD, board-certified ob-gyn and internationally recognized author of multiple trailblazing books, including *Women's Bodies, Women's Wisdom* and *The Wisdom of Menopause*, and Robin McGraw, author of *What's Age Got to Do with It?* Women across America took note and called their doctors. Those doctors pooh-poohing BHRT soon discovered once-loyal patients hanging up and dialing a doctor who would listen.

How to Avoid a
Thelma and Louise–style Plunge

We have now firmly established that with age, hormone levels shift and decline. This does not happen in one fell swoop. It takes years and sometimes decades. Without help, you set yourself up to be a living metaphor of Whack a Mole. If you do not frequent a Chuck E. Cheese pizza parlor, you may not know this game. Here's how it's played: A child holds a mallet over a tabletop with multiple holes the size of a large coffee can. When the motorized mole pops up through a hole, the child squeals, attempting to slam its head. If the mallet hits the mole, the child scores a point. The metaphor: Age is the mallet. Without the right mix of the right kinds of hormones, you are the mole. BHRT can be your escape from this fiendish cycle.

BHRT is a personalized medical approach to restoring optimum hormone balance. Specimens of saliva, blood, or urine can be analyzed to determine exactly which hormones you are deficient in. Then, based on your personal hormone level profile, a prescription can be individualized to give you back exactly what you are missing. These one-size-does-NOT-fit-all prescriptions are compounded onsite in a special compounding pharmacy.

Even with BHRT, what works for you today will likely not work for you sometime in the future. Why? Because with age, levels will continue to shift. The following is a synopsis of my personal experience.

I was forty-three when Randy and I met. I knew nothing about BHRT and was skeptical. Since turning forty, I had gained two to three pounds per year, making me ten pounds over my preferred weight. I was also having difficulty sleeping.

Randy tested and analyzed my hormone levels, quickly diagnosing me as "estrogen dominant." He recommended his over-the-counter bioidentical progesterone cream. Within a month, I dropped the extra pounds and was sleeping through the night. I must admit, I was surprised.

At forty-five, my periods had become irregular, my energy low, and I had once again moved my skinny jeans to the back of my closet. More advanced blood analysis determined progesterone levels had dipped even lower. I now needed prescription-strength bioidentical progesterone. I had now also become deficient in estrogen and tes- tosterone, so Randy also prescribed a bioidentical prescription for each. With my new triumvirate of hormones, I thought I would be "fixed" for good.

Wrong.

Three months following my forty-eighth birthday, I morphed up two pant sizes without any change in eating or exercising habits. New blood work analysis diagnosed a kerflooey thyroid system. A prescription for natural thyroid was added to my regimen.

Today, at fifty-three, I no longer have periods, meaning I am officially postmenopausal. Over the last year, forgetfulness has nagged me, and, as my daddy would say, "My get-up-and-go got up and went." Recent hormone level testing identified a pregnenolone deficiency.

"What the heck is pregnenolone?" I asked Randy.

"Pregnenolone is an essential hormone for women of all ages. The average young adult produces about 14 mg per day. As with other hormones, however, pregnenolone production declines with age. At age seventy-five, the body produces about 60 percent less pregneno- lone than it did at age thirty-five. This has led scientists to consider pregnenolone supplementation as a way to turn back the clock on aging and counter the consequences of this dramatic drop in hormone levels."

I now have a bottle of pregnenolone next to my toothpaste and swallow a capsule every morning.

PASSIONATE ABOUT PROGESTERONE

Can you identify one hormone consistently deficient in all women over thirty-five? The answer is progesterone. Like a middle child, this second hormone in your sex hormone trilogy is often overlooked and its importance underestimated. I am passionate about helping women understand the critical importance of bioidentical progesterone supplementation. Here's why:

Progesterone is often called the "feel good" hormone because of its calming, positive effect on moods. It also has a relaxation response that helps you sleep better. Wondering about your always-pooching tummy? Too much estrogen causes abdominal bloating while progesterone is a natural diuretic.

At a cellular level, progesterone does much more for our overall health and well-being. Evocative clinical studies by Drs. Kenna Stephenson and Helene Leonetti give evidence of progesterone's benefit to both heart and bone health. Researchers at Emory University have found a link between progesterone levels and long-term, optimum cognitive functioning.

Most electrifying are the scientific studies investigating progesterone's role in cancer protection. Progesterone balances, or neutralizes, estrogen's propensity to promote cell growth. Unchecked cell growth is a precursor to cancer. Many studies validate how restoring optimum progesterone levels to eliminate an underlying cellular condition of estrogen dominance can have a cancer-protective effect.

If you want to support your body's optimum hormone balance for life, I recommend you consult a medical professional trained in the intricate endocrinology of hormone balance, preferably one board-certified by the American Academy of Antiaging Medicine (A4M).

However, if you do *nothing else*, review all the clinical evidence underscoring the long-term health benefits of progesterone and consider using an over-the-counter bioidentical progesterone cream. Never, ever, ever take any form of estrogen—even bioidentical—without pairing it with bioidentical progesterone.

TRUST YOUR INSTINCTS

When you need a doctor or medical professional skilled in restoring hormone balance, do your due diligence regarding their training and board certifications in age-management medicine, as well as their clinical reputation for patient satisfaction. Ultimately, trust your gut: Is this someone who will listen to you? Is this someone you want on your team?

More advice on finding a medical professional trained and certified in hormone-level analysis, a compounding pharmacy, and a listing of vetted over-the-counter bioidentical progesterone creams are also included in Appendix B.

PART TWO

MORE NATURAL TIPS TO DIAL BACK YOUR AGE

OUR BELLY FLAT PLAN described in Part 1 is a great start to looking and feeling younger. Now I want to help you see and feel more positive impact more quickly. Chapter 6 describes four more belly-blasting secrets (I am betting three out of four of these you are really going to like). Chapter 7 provides a list of super supplements to accelerate weight loss at a cellular level and fill in any remaining nutritional gaps. Chapter 8 explains why what is good for your waist is also great for your face. Chapter 9 reveals why sexually vital women have decisively better quality of life and then gives options for rejuvenating aging private parts, restoring sexual vitality, and tapping into your innate feminine creative energy.

CHAPTER 6

FOUR MORE BELLY-BLASTING SECRETS

YOU LOVE SPENDING TIME WITH your girlfriends, but did you realize the power you have over each other when it comes to your weight? Your chances of being overweight or obese increase half a percent with every friend in your network who is obese, finds a November 2010 study from Harvard. That more than adds up: Your chances of obesity double for every four obese friends you have, say researchers. Even if that friend lives thousands of miles away, your chances of gaining weight still go up, according to a 2007 *New England Journal of Medicine* study. That may be because your perception of being overweight changes—living larger seems acceptable since the heavy person is a friend.

HANG OUT WITH FIT GIRLFRIENDS

Experts believe your fit girlfriend's lifestyle and behaviors sub-consciously rub off on you, but you don't have to ditch overweight friends to lose weight. In fact, research from Oxford finds making a pact to get fit and trim together is a bonus. Once a friend starts to lose weight, you have a greater chance of losing your unwanted pounds as well. According to Holli Thompson, women's health author and founder of NutritionalStyle.com, "Some interesting studies have been released lately about how integrative those gal-pal relationships are and how they affect our size and ultimately our health."

Studies out of Massachusetts Institute of Technology (MIT) confirm that common lifestyle, body weight, and body mass index are consistent in groups of girlfriends. Healthy friends tend to stick together and support one another's healthy lifestyle choices through exercise, better food choices, and even their optimistic outlook. Makes sense, doesn't it?

Harvard University published studies in 2007 confirming that obesity spreads among friends, and that your chances of becoming obese or gaining weight is in large part dependent upon who you're hanging out with. Arizona State University recently went further with Harvard's study and published more findings, investigating three different pathways toward behavior that might attempt to explain this phenomenon. They found the "monkey see, monkey do" behavior to be the strongest; people don't necessarily think about body weight when they make decisions based on what their group of friends is doing. It seems to be very much a pack mentality when it comes to food, which is why you often see people of the same size together.

You've seen that in action. Your friend says, "Forget the diet; I'm diving in for the ribs and chocolate cake." You're pulled. She's doing it—why can't you? You want to have fun too. You find yourself eating more and more, "having fun," and twenty pounds later, wondering what happened.

The MIT study shows that the opposite can be true. Your girl-friends can support you and lift you up to better choices. Use the power of the "monkey see" mentality to make a date with your girl-friends—go for a power walk, check out the local vegetarian restaurant, meet at Barre class, and try not to make it all about the food. You need those girlfriends, and they need you. Realize the importance of their lifestyles and work toward healthier foods and activities for yourself and all your BFFs.

POUR A SMALL GLASS OF WINE

Sadie adjourned her last meeting as Temple board chair by inviting the entire board to lunch. Seated outside at the Sunset Grille, the women kvetched about the latest market tumble, gubernatorial fund-raising, and the pluses and minuses of long-wearing nail polish. Overhearing Sadie request a wine-by-the-glass list, conversation screeched to a halt.

"Celebrating?" Kendra queried, disapproval in her eyebrows.

"Just sticking to my diet," Sadie smiled.

"Your diet?" Neta squealed, tugging at her too-tight knit top.

"Yes, my diet. A few months ago our daughter Amy attended a medical conference in Boston on obesity and health risks. A paper was presented showing that women who were light to moderate drinkers were less likely to gain weight over time. Amy knows how frustrated I've become watching my weight creep up so she e-mailed the link to the study and urged me to give it a try. For two months now I've been having a little bit of wine every day. Without doing anything else different, I'm down eight pounds."

Staying well hydrated catalyzes weight loss and staves off poor brain function, lethargy, and low moods. Water, herbal teas, broth-based soups, low-fat milk, and fresh produce all boost hydration.

Wine, though not hydrating, provides antioxidants and has been clinically correlated with less weight gain for women as they age. As stated earlier, Randy and most doctors agree that, a "splash of wine" is a healthful component of our Belly Flat Diet. Studies back them up: In 2010 researchers at Brigham and Women's Hospital in Boston published the first long-term study on women's drinking habits and weight gain. The study involved 19,220 women over the age of thirty-eight who were of normal weight. After thirteen years, women who consistently consumed a moderate amount of alcohol per day were 30 percent less likely to be overweight and nearly 70 percent less likely to be obese than nondrinkers.

Once again, there's a hormone connection. The relationship between alcohol consumption and insulin resistance evidences a U-shaped curve: insulin resistance was shown to be minimal in women with regular mild to moderate (3 oz.) alcohol consumption and higher in both heavy drinkers and women who never had a drink.

Finally, for ladies loving the vine, a weight loss solution to toast!

EAT SOME CHOCOLATE

A 2012 study found that people who frequently ate chocolate had a lower body mass index (BMI) than people who didn't. Is it time to ditch fat-free for fudge?

For the study, published in the March 26 issue of *Archives of Internal Medicine*, researchers examined more than one thousand healthy men and women who were free of heart disease, diabetes, and cholesterol problems. They were all enrolled in another study that measured the effects of cholesterol-lowering statin drugs, but for this study researchers assigned them questionnaires that gauged how often participants chowed down on chocolate.

The researchers found that the participants—who were an average age of fifty-seven—ate chocolate an average of twice a week and exercised roughly 3.5 times per week. But the more frequent chocolate-eaters had smaller BMIs, a ratio of height and weight that's used to measure obesity.

What explains the effect? Even though chocolate can be loaded with calories, it's full of antioxidants and other ingredients that may promote weight loss. Research also shows that a little bit of chocolate can be good for your health. Compared with people who rarely ate chocolate (about one bar per month), the people who ate the most chocolate (slightly more than one bar per week) had a 27 percent and 48 percent reduced risk of heart attack and stroke, respectively.

Please don't read this section and believe I am giving you carte blanche to eat a chocolate bar a day. As with the recommendation on wine, the key is moderation, but researchers' definition of "moderation" can vary. After reviewing the scientific literature and clinical studies, Randy recommends an average amount of 6.7 grams of chocolate per day, corresponding to a small square of chocolate twice or three times a week.

CHEW

Dr. Pam Rama is a superb cardiologist who has risen to the zenith of her career as the medical director of Baptist Health System's HeartWise program while also raising four children. I don't think I could tie her shoelaces. Add that to the fact that she is drop-dead gorgeous, and it would be easy to be intimidated, except she is down-to-earth and fun.

When we scheduled dinner to talk about this book, I didn't realize until the menu was in my hands that I would be intimidated about what to order when eating with my cardiologist. I chose a green salad, grilled salmon, and steamed broccoli.

Actually, I thought, *that is exactly what I would have ordered anyway.*

Our food arrived. I took a couple of bites, still chatting away. Pam stopped me.

"Chew."

"Huh?"

"Chew more. Chew each bite at least thirty times, forty is better."

"Really?" I responded, imagining with this new directive we could be at the restaurant until dawn. "Why?"

"New research shows chewing to have many health benefits, including weight control. Check it out."

Researchers from Iowa State University (ISU) presented findings at April 2012's Experimental Biology Conference demonstrating that Dr. Rama's tip of taking your time by chewing longer and slower during a meal really can help you eat less. This weight loss tip is based on the fact that the longer you chew, the more the hunger hormone, called ghrelin, is suppressed, while another hormone, called leptin, whose role is to stimulate feelings of fullness, increases.

In the study, twenty ISU students were given a metronome and told to chew every time it ticked. The students were divided into two groups where the metronome ticked for fifteen times with one group and forty times with the other group before the two groups were allowed to swallow their chewed food. During the study, plasma glucose and hormone levels were measured, as well as the students' sense of appetite. What the researchers discovered was that the students who chewed more actually ate less than the students who chewed less.

"When people chewed the pizza forty times before swallowing, there was a reduction in hunger, preoccupation with food, and a desire to eat," said James Hollis, an Iowa State assistant professor of food science and human nutrition who coauthored the study.

The reason why chewing longer is healthier is this: The longer you chew your food, the more the food will be exposed to saliva, and as a result more nutrients will be absorbed. This is especially true for nuts and seeds, as well as fruits and vegetables, as they contain hard cellulose fibers that cannot be broken down anywhere but in the mouth. This is why when you eat nuts, corn, or other vegetables, they just seem to pass through your system if they are not properly chewed.

When your body is able to absorb all the nutrients from the foods that you eat, you will have much higher energy levels. On top of that, no energy will be wasted on eliminating foods that the body cannot digest or break down.

CHAPTER 7

SUPER SUPPLEMENTS

I N CAGES AT MCMASTER UNIVERSITY in Hamilton, Ontario, sits a group of mice who don't act their age. Unbelievably, they don't seem to be aging at all. For several years, the Canadian mice have been drinking a cocktail of thirty dietary supplements and vitamins. The concoction seems to be keeping the rodents young.

Scientists say the mice that were given the anti-aging cocktail had an unusual spring in their step. They had no loss of physical activity compared to a group of mice who didn't imbibe. In fact, those mice showed a 50 percent decrease in physical activity. Astonishingly, the combination of vitamins and supplements lengthened the life span of the rodents that took it by 11 percent. Did the Canadian scientists discover the legendary Fountain of Youth? If you are a mouse, they did.

Forget the mice, what about us girls? Can certain supplements keep us healthier? Can swallowing some pill truly help balance our hormones? Is there solid medical science to validate how nutritional supplements slow down or reverse our aging, or could our health and wallets be preyed upon by some vitamin and supplement manufacturer promising to turn back our inner clock?

"Yes" is the correct response to all the questions above. Succinctly, yes, there is solid medical science to support the benefits of nutritional supplementation—and yes, you could easily spend way too much money on anti-aging supplements that provide no true health benefits. This chapter provides a framework to help you sort through the hype and clutter to help you make your best informed choice about whether or not supplements are right for you.

WHO NEEDS SUPPLEMENTS?

"In an ideal world, no one would need dietary supplements," says Randy. "Our Belly Flat Diet would provide all the vitamins, minerals, and nutrients your body needs no matter your age. Unfortunately, even women who do their best to 'eat right' will likely need some nutritional supplementation, because with age our bodies lose the ability to metabolize and store needed nutrients."

Statistics indicate that dietary supplement use is widespread among US adults age twenty and older. The percentage of the US population who use at least one dietary supplement increased from 42 percent in 1988–94 to 53 percent in 2003–6 (Figure 1). Women were found to be more likely to use one or more dietary supplements than men. More recent industry survey results, many of which point to usage in 2011, settle around the 70 percent mark. Vitamins and dietary supplements (VDS) enjoy broad acceptance in the United States, where nearly half of all users reported using more than one supplement daily, and nearly 10 percent took five or more supplements a day.

Figure 1. Trends in the percentage of persons using dietary supplements, by gender for adults aged 20 and over; United States, 1988–2006

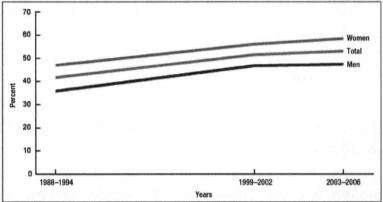

NOTES: Significant linear trend from 1988–1994 through 2003–2006. Statistically significant difference for men compared with women for all time periods, $p \leq 0.05$ for comparison between genders within survey periods. Age adjusted by direct method to the year 2000 projected U.S. population.
SOURCE; CDC/NCHS, National Health and Nutrition Examination Surveys.

One might argue that the growing trend of supplement use is a result of a baby-boomer consumer-driven frenzy to ward off the Grim Reaper, but guess what? Odds are, like Randy, your doctor and nurse are not betting on the food on the table to provide all the nutrients he or she needs.

An online survey administered in October 2007 to 900 physicians and 277 nurses by Ipsos Public Affairs for the Council for Responsible Nutrition (CRN), a trade association representing the dietary supplement industry, found that 72 percent of physicians and 89 percent of nurses used dietary supplements regularly, occasionally, or seasonally. Regular use of dietary supplements was reported by 51 percent of physicians and 59 percent of nurses.

The most common reason given for using dietary supplements was for overall health and wellness (40 percent of physicians and 48 percent of nurses), but more than two-thirds cited more than one reason for using the products. When asked whether they "ever recommend dietary supplements" to their patients, 79 percent of physicians and 82 percent of nurses said they did. Also, almost all said they recommend supplements to their patients, whether or not they took them themselves.

MELT BELLY FAT MORE QUICKLY

Drawing on his original training as a compounding pharmacist specializing in pharmacognosy (plant-based medicine), Randy continuously researches and tests hordes of nutritional supplements to ascertain their true mechanism for influencing estrogen metabolism. In concert with our Belly Flat Diet, he recommends a select group of supplements that he has found to expedite the elimination of too much circulating estrogen, thereby enhancing healthy hormone balance and promoting weight loss and weight management more quickly. They are:

Calcium D-Glucarate

Calcium D-glucarate is a natural substance that promotes the body's detoxification process and supports hormonal balance. Calcium D-glucarate facilitates the detoxification process by inhibiting the reabsorption of estrogen-like toxins into the bloodstream, allowing them to leave the body and be excreted in the feces. In animals, calcium D-glucarate has been found to lower unhealthy estrogen levels and thereby inhibit the development or progression of cancer.

Diindolymethane (DIM)

DIM is a phytonutrient akin to the indole-3-carbinol (I3C) found in cruciferous vegetables. DIM has unique hormonal benefits. It supports the activity of enzymes that improve estrogen metabolism. DIM helps support PMS symptoms, fat loss, and healthy estrogen metabolism.

The B Vitamins

The B vitamins, such as B_1, B_2, B_3, B_5, B_6, B_{12}, and folate, do a lot within your body to support estrogen detoxification. Conversely, if your body is deficient in B vitamins, you will have higher levels of circulating estrogens. By now, you definitely know that increased estrogen levels lead to estrogen dominance, and estrogen dominance will most certainly lead to weight gain and the inability to get that weight off.

B vitamins also impact estrogen activity for the hormone receptors at the cellular level. Clinical studies have shown that high levels of intracellular (e.g., within the cell) B_6 can decrease the binding response at the estrogen hormone receptor site. What happens at the cellular level is sort of like an internal game of musical chairs: if the music stops and B_6 sits down in the "estrogen chair," then the estrogen molecule is out of the game.

Vitamin B complex supplements also may help with a variety of health conditions, including anxiety, depression, fatigue, heart disease, premenstrual syndrome, and skin problems. In addition, many people take a vitamin B complex to increase energy, enhance mood, improve memory, and stimulate the immune system.

Because the B vitamins work together to perform such vital tasks at the cellular level, Randy recommends you take the entire B complex, not just one or two of the B vitamins.

Vitamin E

Vitamin E has been shown to reduce PMS-related breast tenderness, nervousness, depression, headache, fatigue, and insomnia. Low vitamin E levels were linked to estrogen dominance. Furthermore, vitamin E deficiency has been found to inhibit estrogen detoxification.

Calcium-Magnesium Combo

Magnesium is another supplement that helps the body eliminate excess estrogen. For women, magnesium levels tend to fall at certain times during the menstrual cycle. These shifts in magnesium levels can upset an optimum calcium-magnesium ratio. In proper balance, the body better absorbs and assimilates the calcium it needs and allows calcium to migrate out of tissue and organs where it doesn't belong.

Without magnesium, calcium may not be fully utilized. Underabsorption of calcium can lead to menstrual cramps. Similar to a vitamin E deficiency, when the body does not have enough magnesium to support calcium absorption, many women report PMS symptoms, such as mood swings, fatigue, headaches, and sleeplessness.

Premenstrual chocolate craving is a phenomenon that has puzzled a great many physicians. They have been unable to explain why some women have this overwhelming urge to eat lots and lots of chocolate right before their periods, yet at other times of the month, their chocolate cravings remain under control. Women find their PMS-related chocolate cravings abate when taking a calcium-magnesium combo.

7- Keto Dehydroepiandrosterone (DHEA)

Dehydroepiandrosterone (DHEA) is one of the hormones pro-duced by the adrenal glands. After being secreted, it circulates in the bloodstream as DHEA-sulfate (DHEAS) and is converted as needed into other hormones. Since it is a precursor to testosterone, DHEA may help build muscle. It is very unusual for anyone under the age of thirty-five or forty to have low DHEA levels. As we age, however, the body's production of DHEA declines, so people older than forty can most definitely become DHEA deficient.

While many anti-aging enthusiasts are familiar with DHEA, far fewer are likely to be as aware of its metabolite, 7-Keto DHEA, which functions within the body to safely boost immune function and help reduce body fat. The term 7-Keto DHEA is, in fact, a brand name for the chemical compound 3-acetyl-7-dehydroepiandrosterone. Human blood levels of both 7-Keto DHEA and DHEA tend to rise and fall in a similar pattern with age: increasing until the twenties, beginning to decline in the thirties, and continuing to decline until the levels are reduced by about 50 percent by age fifty. Clinical stud-ies have shown that as 7-Keto DHEA levels go down in middle age, body weight tends to go up.

7-Keto DHEA stimulates weight loss through a process called thermogenesis. This term refers to the creation of heat at a cellular level. The more thermogenesis, the higher the metabolic rate and the more fat that is literally burned up as energy. Studies have also dem-onstrated that 7-Keto does not accumulate in the body over time and is free of unhealthy side effects.

Because 7-Keto DHEA is a natural hormone metabolite, it bene-fits the body in two ways: (1) it helps restore hormone balance while, at the same time, it (2) works internally to melt away those unwanted pounds.

Chitosan

Chitosan is processed from the shells of crustaceans such as shrimp, lobster, and crabs. Basically stated, chitosan acts as a superfiber. The swelling action of chitosan creates a sensation of feeling full, thereby serving to suppress the appetite. In addition, the superfiber characteristics of chitosan foster a natural cleansing process that is extremely vital to weight loss.

Chitosan is also able to absorb between six and ten times its weight in fat and oils. It then converts the fat molecules into a form that the human body does not absorb. When chitosan causes less fat to enter the body, the body has to turn to previously stored body fat to burn for energy. The net result: weight loss.

Six Vitamins and Supplements to Support Hormone Balance

Calcium D-glucarate: Take 1,000 mg twice per day

Diindolymethajne (DIM): Take 200 mg per day

B-Complex: Take 1 capsule per day

Vitamin E: Take 400 IU per day

Calcium-magnesium combo: Take a ratio of two parts calcium (1,400 mg) to one part magnesium (750 mg)

7-Keto DHEA: Take 100 mg per day

Chitosan: Take 750 mg three times a day

EVERY WOMAN ALSO NEEDS . . .

I take more than a dozen supplements a day. That sounds like a lot to swallow, but my approach to nutritional supplementation is not hit or miss. I rely on my team of physician experts—Randy and Drs. Lori Leaseburge and Pam Rama for guidance. Their shared medical opinion is that every woman older than thirty-five should also take the following supplements:

Multivitamin

The Harvard School of Public Health suggests a daily multivitamin, calling it a "great nutrition insurance policy." But what about the *Wall Street Journal* article "Study Finds Multivitamins Don't Cut Risk of Heart Attack" (November 5, 2012)?

"No single pill should be intended to replace diet and exercise," says Dr. Leaseburge. "There is no magic bullet, but a good multivitamin will help even out the ups and downs of women's sometime irregular diet and lifestyle habits. And, with regard to that article and the studies cited within, I would question the quality of the multivitamin used in the study."

Not all vitamins are manufactured equally (see more on how to choose quality supplements in the pages that follow).

Vitamin D

According to Randy, "Most people—and even their physicians— are unaware of the important role that vitamin D plays in retarding aging, promoting energy and health weight maintenance, boosting the immune system, and reducing your risk of cancer. And, unfortunately, most people are unaware that their body is deficient in needed vitamin D levels. Though vitamin D is naturally produced by the human body when exposed to sunlight, most American adults spend most of their time indoors, and when they are outside, they usually wear sunscreen. Even though my medical practice is in the sunny state of Florida, I routinely test my patients' vitamin D levels."

Randy is not alone in his medical opinion. Dr. Oz states that "it is commonly believed that over 50 percent of Americans are vitamin D deficient." When unrecognized and untreated, vitamin D deficiency can lead to more serious conditions, including osteoporosis, high blood pressure, heart and inflammatory problems, multiple sclerosis, and chronic pain, among others.

CoQ_{10}

Our bodies produce CoQ_{10}, a substance that's necessary for cells to function. It helps produce an important molecule known as adenosine triphosphate, or ATP. ATP is the fuel that helps power the energy-producing center of the cell known as mitochondria. As we get older, our body produces less CoQ_{10}, and as a result, our cells don't function as they should. According to the Mayo Clinic, those who suffer from chronic diseases such as Parkinson's, cancer, diabetes, and cardiovascular disease have lower CoQ_{10} levels than healthy people.

Researchers also believe that taking CoQ_{10} as a supplement can help prevent heart disease. It helps prevent blood from clotting and may act as an antioxidant, which protects our cells against the effects of free radicals that can damage cells and cause heart disease. Moreover, researchers suspect CoQ_{10} supplements may improve the health of diabetics by managing blood sugar, cholesterol, and blood pressure.

Omega-3 Fish Oil

Fish oil helps reduce internal inflammation in the body. According to the American Heart Association, omega-3 fatty acids decrease cardiac arrhythmias, reduce risk of sudden heart attack, and lower blood pressure, triglycerides, and cholesterol levels. The essential omega-3 fatty acids help to alleviate pain, depression, and uterine cramps and pain at the onset of menstruation. One of the main causes of PMS appears to be excess production of pro-inflammatory eicosanoids. Fish oil contains high quantities of eicosapentaenoic acid (EPA), which helps the body produce anti-inflammatory eicosanoids, providing relief.

Omega-3 fish oil helps to energize and hydrate cells of the body, adding shine, gloss, and health to skin and hair. It also protects the skin against the harmful ultraviolet rays of the sun. Consumption of omega-3 fish oil has also been found to act as a stimulant for hair growth.

When patients complain of burping up a fishy taste when taking fish oil supplements, Dr. Rama says, "Store them in your freezer. The temperature won't change your ability to swallow or digest them, but the fishy taste goes away."

Probiotics

Probiotic products contain bacteria and/or yeasts that assist in restoring the balance in our gut. Probiotics are believed to protect us in two ways. The first is the role that they play in our digestive tract. We know that our digestive tract needs a healthy balance between the good and bad bacteria, so what gets in the way of this? It looks like our lifestyle is both the problem and the solution. Poor food choices, emotional stress, lack of sleep, antibiotic overuse, other drugs, and environmental influences can all shift the balance in favor of the bad bacteria.

When the digestive tract is healthy, it filters out and eliminates things that can damage it, such as harmful bacteria, toxins, chemicals, and other waste products. On the flip side, it takes in the things that our body needs (nutrients from food and water) and absorbs and helps deliver them to the cells where they are needed.

The idea is not to kill off all of the bad bacteria. Our body needs both bad and good bacteria. The problem occurs when the balance is shifted and we have more bad than good. An imbalance has been associated with diarrhea, urinary tract infections, muscle pain, and fatigue.

The other way that probiotics help is the impact that they have on our immune system. Some physicians believe that this role is the most important. Our immune system is our protection against germs. When it doesn't function properly, we can suffer from allergic reactions, autoimmune disorders (for example, ulcerative colitis, Crohn's disease, and rheumatoid arthritis), and infections (for example, infectious diarrhea, *Helicobacter pylori*, skin infections, and vaginal infections).

CAUTION: BE CERTAIN OF QUALITY

Dietary supplements are regulated by the FDA, but not as drugs or as foods. The rules for dietary supplements are as follows: Manufacturers don't have to seek FDA approval before putting dietary supplements on the market. In addition, companies can claim that products address a nutrient deficiency, support health, or are linked to body functions—if they have supporting research and they include a disclaimer that the FDA hasn't evaluated the claim.

Manufacturers must follow good manufacturing practices to ensure that supplements are processed consistently and meet quality standards. These regulations are intended to keep the wrong ingredients and contaminants, such as pesticides and lead, out of supplements, as well as make sure that the right ingredients are included in appropriate amounts.

Once a dietary supplement is on the market, the FDA is responsible for monitoring its safety. If the FDA finds a product to be unsafe, it can take action against the manufacturer or distributor or both, and it may issue a warning or require that the product be removed from the market.

These regulations provide assurance that dietary supplements meet certain quality standards and that the FDA can intervene to remove dangerous products from the market. The rules do not, however, guarantee that supplements are safe for everyone. Because many supplements contain active ingredients that have strong effects in the body, these products can pose unexpected risks. For example, taking a combination of herbal supplements or using supplements together with prescribed medications could lead to harmful, even life-threatening results. For this reason, it's important to talk with your doctor about the supplements you intend to take.

And not all supplements are of equal quality. Manufacturers of supplements are responsible for ensuring that the claims they make about their products aren't false or misleading and that they're backed up by adequate evidence. However, they aren't required to submit this evidence to the FDA.

According to Randy, "Supplement manufacturers often add in a variety of fillers to their vitamin and mineral supplements for numerous reasons: easier and faster production, colorants to make products more eye-appealing, coatings to make pills and capsules easier to swallow. The reasons for using fillers aside, the real problem lies in how these fillers impact your body and health. Simply put, it's not good. Just as processed foods are loaded with additives and fillers, the same goes for vitamins. Any supplement that has additives and fillers may be harmful to your health in the same way those processed foods are. Some unhealthy fillers include hydrogenated oils, artificial colors, and magnesium stearate, which is used as a lubricant so that the vitamins don't stick to one another or the equipment being used. The controversy surrounds a few studies on magnesium stearate. One study links this compound to creating a suppressed immune system. Other studies show that this 'chalk' creates a biofilm in the body. This biofilm blocks the body from absorbing any of the needed nutrients. Titanium oxide is another filler widely used as a pigment in vitamins. However, the research is now showing that exposure to this metal (along with other metals) can lead to problems with the immune function in the body."

HOW DO YOU CHOOSE?

When it comes to choosing which and what brand of supplement, I want you to be a smart consumer and do your homework. Don't just rely on a product's marketing. Look for objective, research-based information to evaluate any health or medical claims. To get reliable information about a particular supplement, I recommend you:

- Ask your doctor or pharmacist. Even if they don't know about a specific supplement, they may be able to point you to the latest medical guidance about its uses and risks. Today there are proven higher-quality supplement companies whose integrity is enhanced because they choose to only be sold through medical professional offices. We offer Randy's signature brand in our National Medicine Pharmacy and on our website, www.agelessandwellness.com. Metagenics, Xymogen, and OrthoMolecular brands are three others in this league.

- Look for scientific research findings. Two good sources include the National Center for Complementary and Alternative Medicine (NCCAM) and the Office of Dietary Supplements. Both have websites that provide information to help consumers make informed choices about dietary supplements.

- Contact the manufacturer. If you have questions about a specific product, call the manufacturer or distributor. Ask to talk with someone who can answer questions, such as what data the company has to substantiate its products' claims.

CHAPTER 8

WHAT'S GOOD FOR YOUR WAIST IS GREAT FOR YOUR FACE

M Y GRANDMOTHER USED TO SAY that a smiling, kind, and well-mannered woman will dazzle no matter the age or shape of her features. Good news: That truism did not go out with hats and gloves. When I consider all the women interviewed for this book, the one that stands out to me as hands-down most beautiful is Susan Eister Estes of Richmond, Virginia. A glorious blond with an enigmatic smile and ready laugh, Susan will likely continue turning heads no matter her age. What makes Susan's beauty especially astonishing, however, is that she maintains such a countenance while devotedly caring for a husband with Alzheimer's disease in their home.

"I try to never feel sorry for myself or slump around," says Susan. "I get up, get dressed, get busy and always put on lipstick."

But, as we age, we may need more than a great smile and bright tube of lipstick to look our prettiest. Good news: our Belly Flat Plan will not only help you lose those pounds and have more energy, it can help turn back the clock on your face! Here's how:

BELLY FLAT DIET
REJUVENATES YOUR FACE

A study published in March 2010 in the *Journal of the American Academy of Dermatology* supports the idea that certain vitamins help to protect our skin. Better yet, many of the same foods that can boost your defenses against skin cancer (the most common type of cancer) will also help keep your skin looking younger and smoother and ward off wrinkles. Our bonus: they are all belly-blaster foods! Here's how they promote youthful beauty from the inside out:

Vitamin C–Rich Foods

In 2007, research published in the *American Journal of Clinical Nutrition* showed that eating more vitamin C–rich foods, such as citrus fruits, strawberries, broccoli, and red peppers, may help ward off wrinkles and age-related dryness. Vitamin C's skin-smoothing effects may be due to its ability to mop up free radicals produced from ultraviolet rays and also its role in collagen synthesis. Collagen is fibrous protein that keeps skin firm, and vitamin C is essential for collagen production.

Pink grapefruit is a vitamin C–rich, super skin-beautifying food. Pink grapefruit gets its pink-red hue from lycopene, a carotenoid that may help to keep your skin smooth. In a study published in 2008 in the *European Journal of Pharmaceutics and Biopharmaceutics,* researchers found that of the twenty individuals studied, those who had higher skin concentrations of lycopene had smoother skin.

Omega-3-Rich Fatty Fish

Omega-3-rich fish may help keep your skin looking youthful and prevent skin cancer. The omega-3 fatty acids DHA and EPA (docosahexaenoic and eicosapentaenoic acids, respectively) found in salmon, tuna, sardines, and mackerel may shield cell walls from free-radical damage caused by UV rays, according to a 2009 study in the *American Journal of Clinical Nutrition*. Researchers followed the eating habits of more than 1,100 Australian adults for approximately five years and found that for those who ate a little more than 5 ounces of omega-3-rich fish (such as salmon) each week, the development of precancerous skin lesions decreased by almost 30 percent.

EPA has been shown to preserve collagen, a fibrous protein that keeps skin firm. EPA in combination with DHA helps to prevent skin cancer by reducing inflammatory compounds that can promote tumor growth, according to Homer S. Black, PhD, professor emeritus in the Department of Dermatology at Baylor College of Medicine in Houston.

Whole Grains

Whole-grain bread, pasta, and cereal are surprisingly high in antioxidants (whole-wheat cereal, for example, contains a comparable amount to most fruits and vegetables), and eating additional antioxidants is key to youth-proofing your complexion, says Lisa Drayer, RD. "The levels of the body's natural antioxidants decrease with age, so adding them to your diet becomes even more important."

Almonds

Eating a handful of almonds (a one-ounce serving is about 20 to 24 whole nuts) every day boosts levels of vitamin E, one of the most important antioxidants for skin health.

Red Wine and Dark Chocolate

The magic effect red wine and dark chocolate can have on our skin comes from antioxidants. The dark skin and seeds of the grapes in red wine are rich in polyphenols, a type of antioxidant that includes resveratrol. The antioxidants in red wine soak up damaging free radicals that play a role in aging. Dark chocolate also has a high concentration of polyphenols and provides the same benefits of protecting cell membranes with anti-inflammatory properties.

CONSIDER FARM TO FACE

We've talked about why you should choose organic foods when possible and, also, the importance of detoxing your home from chemicals that can silently sabotage your health while accelerating your aging and putting children at risk for precocious puberty. Now consider the potential benefits of 100 percent natural skin care.

While the previously quoted statistics linking petrochemicals in common skin care and beauty products are disturbing, I must admit I have personally struggled for years to find an organic skin-care line that not only feels and smells good but works to decrease lines and signs of aging. My good news is that today there are a growing number of excellent organic lines on the market with dynamic women leading this skin-care revolution. Several excellent companies are listed in Appendix B, but here I want to give a shout-out to two women who started their companies motivated by personal experience.

Kelly Teegarden created her organic line after a long struggle to regain her health after a near-terminal bout of thyroid cancer. Kelly says, "I am convinced that Kelly Teegarden Organics (KTO) is my 'why' for getting cancer. I thank God I am still here to help as many people as I can on their crusade to health." KTO products are available online and at Whole Foods.

Similarly, while pregnant and helping care for her stepfather with cancer, Tata Harper determined to do everything she could to keep toxic petrochemicals out of her beauty regimen. "Beauty was and is a priority for me, but health is an even bigger one. Nevertheless, I did not think women like me should have to sacrifice one for the other."

Tata drew from her training as an industrial engineer to work with a team of chemists, biologists, botanists, agriculturists, and aromatherapists from around the globe to create her proprietary 100 percent natural products.

Tata says, "Beauty is a way of living, not a product. What a woman puts on her face and the skin of her body should match who she is on the inside, as well as how she chooses to live. If our eyes are the mirrors of our souls, then our faces and skin are a reflection of our choices. Why wouldn't every woman choose natural, healthy skincare products that can help increase our visible beauty versus those that can make us sick? Why wouldn't we make natural beauty an inside-out nonnegotiable priority?"

Exercise Helps You Look Younger

"Anything that promotes healthy circulation also helps keep your skin healthy and vibrant," says dermatologist Ellen Marmur, MD, author of *Simple Skin Beauty: Every Woman's Guide to a Lifetime of Healthy, Gorgeous Skin* and associate professor of dermatology at Mount Sinai School of Medicine. By increasing blood flow, exercise helps nourish skin cells and keep them vital.

"Blood carries oxygen and nutrients to working cells throughout the body, including the skin," says Marmur. "In addition to providing oxygen, blood flow also helps carry away waste products, including free radicals, from working cells. Contrary to some claims, exercise doesn't detoxify the skin. The job of neutralizing toxins belongs mostly to the liver. But by increasing blood flow, a bout of exercise helps flush cellular debris out of the system. You can think of it as cleansing your skin from the inside."

The boost in blood flow and oxygen to the skin cells also carries nutrients that improve skin health. Also, when you exercise, your skin begins to produce more of its natural oils, which helps skin look supple and healthy.

GET MORE BEAUTY REST

Most people have experienced sallow skin and puffy eyes after a few nights of missed sleep. But it turns out that chronic sleep loss can lead to lackluster skin, fine lines, and dark circles under the eyes. When you don't get enough sleep, your body releases more of the stress hormone cortisol. In excess amounts, cortisol can break down skin collagen, the protein that keeps skin smooth and elastic.

A person may look a decade older in response to *stress-induced* changes in facial tissues that often accompany insomnia. Few people are aware, however, that chronic insomnia inflicts significant damage to skin tissues, from premature aging to disorders like eczema, psoriasis, and atopic dermatitis.

Lack of sleep also upsets the balance of two more hormones: ghrelin and leptin. When you sleep less than eight hours, ghrelin levels go up and leptin levels go down. Ghrelin is the hormone that makes you feel hungry while leptin signals the brain that you are full. Sleep-deprived women frequently say, "I am hungry all the time," but their drive to eat has nothing to do with a big appetite or weak willpower and everything to do with their hormones.

CHAPTER 9

Pump Up
Your Pelvic Power

AGING RESEARCH INDICATES sexually vital women have decisively better quality of life indicators and self-report a more positive aging experience. Many women make the mistake of equating sexual vitality to sexual activity and carnal mirth, particularly intercourse. Don't! No matter your age, sexual vitality is our inner, God-given energizer for joy and creative juiciness. If you have fun in the sack, enjoy the bonus while burning the calories.

Multiple factors dim sexual vitality and dampen creative juiciness, including aging private parts. The good news: we can fix those.

When There's a Drought Down There

Mary Nell parked her car across the street and looked in the rearview mirror, making certain her hat, scarf, and sunglasses obscured most of her face, then took a deep breath to wind up her courage. A few years back, she would never have imagined stepping into a shop that sold adult movies and sex toys, but she was desperate. Intercourse had become painful, often with skin tearing and bleeding. She had embarrassingly bought a lubricant from the drugstore, but it itched and burned, and the day after using it, she woke up with a nasty urinary tract infection. That night Nigel began sleeping in the guest room down the hall.

Ironically, the next week Pastor Duncan asked her and Nigel to host a small group of five couples in their home every Wednesday. "I can think of no better twosome to lead this six-session video-based study on how intimacy in marriage is part of God's plan. Nigel and Mary Nell, will you do it?"

Mary Nell wasn't sure if God looked less favorably on hypocrites or loose women, but crossing the street and walking into a store with a purple neon penis in its window, she felt like both.

Lack of vaginal moisture and lubrication does not mean you are entering the life stage of the dried-up crone, nor does it correlate to lack of love or lust. If your vagina is so dry that intercourse is uncomfortable or painful, no lingerie, sexy video, hours of foreplay, or amount of prayer or meditation will get your juices flowing.

Vaginal dryness is more common for perimenopausal and menopausal women but is often a surprising and depressing issue for younger, regularly menstruating women. Studies cited by the National Institutes of Health also show that, because estrogen levels fall after childbirth and remain suppressed while breastfeeding, vaginal dryness can be a problem for new moms. Also, women with premature ovarian failure, polycystic ovarian syndrome (PCOS), vulvar dystrophy (a condition where the outer part of the vagina becomes dry and the skin thickens) and vulvodinyia (a condition where there is pain around the opening of the vagina where there is no identifiable cause) are at risk.

And if you think vaginal dryness is an issue for only the sexually active, think again. Women not having intercourse or engaging in manual or oral stimulation of the genital area often complain of vaginal dryness. Some say the soreness, burning, and itching makes them uncomfortable sitting, standing, exercising, or urinating.

If your vagina is as dry as an emery board, stop feeling damaged or just plain old. Evaluate recommended lifestyle changes and potential treatment options, and work with a knowledgeable medical professional as needed. Tips for improving vaginal lubrication include:

Replace what's missing: Synergistic bioidentical estrogen, progesterone, and/or testosterone replacement can reinvigorate and nourish fragile vaginal tissue.

Clean up carefully: Certain personal hygiene products, such as soaps, bubble baths, deodorants, and even douching with water, can contribute to vaginal dryness.

Wake up your clitoris: Arousal stimulates lubrication; however, a woman's clitoris (her primary genital organ of arousal) can become less sensitive with age, hormonal changes, or the aftereffects of a hysterectomy. Wake up your clitoris by embracing the miracle of masturbation. If you enjoy some variety, a vibrator can also be very handy. Good news for the accessory-loving diva: vibrators come in a variety of styles and colors. (Check out the Deluxe Rabbit Pearl Vibrator in pink.)

Play with toys: The vaginal wall can atrophy (weaken), causing foreplay and intercourse to become uncomfortable to painful.

Try a sex toy such as a vaginal dilator or dildo to increase the diameter of your vagina.

Add foreign moisture wisely: Over-the-counter lubricants may be helpful, but read the labels before you buy. For instance, there is a difference between a lubricant to increase vulvo-vaginal comfort and a vaginal moisturizer hydrating the mucous membrane lining of the vaginal canal. Also, some ingredients in certain over-the-counter products are absolute no-no's because they create a medium for bacteria transfer and growth, thereby increasing risk of urinary tract infection. Recommended resources for over-the-counter lubricants are included in Appendix B.

URINE IS NEVER AN ATTRACTIVE ACCESSORY

Four blocks into her walk, Terri stopped, cagily adjusted her underwear under dark, baggy sweat pants, then sighed and turned home. Despite an absorbent liner, her panties were dangerously damp. Continuing around the golf course would, at best, mean uncomfortable chafing and, at worst, a full-fledged accident before she reached the clubhouse just six blocks down on her carefully mapped-out route of accessible restrooms. Tears seeped under her sunglasses.

Walking four miles with my neighborhood gang used to be my favorite part of the day, she cried inside. *Now even walking alone risks humiliation. This bathroom business is ruining my life. I'm afraid to go to church or a basketball game with Thomas. What if I leak and people around me smell pee pee? And when it comes to sex, Thomas has been patient, but how long can that last?*

Urine is unattractive, and damp panties are uncomfortable. Still, one in six women experience overactive bladder (OAB). While more common in older adults, OAB can strike women of all ages. For women like Terri, OAB puts the brakes on a great deal of joy and quality of life. But it doesn't have to be this way.

Did you know that there is more than one kind of leaky bladder? "Stress incontinence" is when small amounts of urine escape when you sneeze, pee, laugh, or exert pressure on the bladder by lifting or exercising. "Urge incontinence" is when you *have to go now* and urine escapes before you reach the toilet.

Why urine leakage happens during sex is easy enough to understand. Sexual activity can place extra pressure on the abdomen, causing urine to leak. This causes many women to avoid sex, as it makes them feel unclean or unattractive. Women suffering from stress incontinence usually can tell when during intercourse they are most likely to leak. But urge incontinence occurs unpredictably, making it difficult to feel sensual and/or fully enjoy sex. The chance of embarrassment is also greater—much more urine leaks during an episode of urge incontinence compared with stress incontinence, and women with urge incontinence often leak during orgasm.

Whichever type of incontinence you might suffer, an integrated approach can help get you out of the bathroom sans the absorbent pads in your panties. New surgical techniques (bladder slings, bladder neck suspension, the injection of bulking agents such as collagen, or sacral nerve stimulation via a small, pacemakerlike device surgically placed under the skin) may very well give you back your life. Before you make that decision to go under anesthesia, talk with your doctor about nonsurgical approaches, including physical therapy and pelvic-floor yoga exercises.

You and your doctor have most likely heard how Kegel exercises help strengthen the pelvic floor. I would wager that neither you nor your doctor knows that the National Institutes of Health recognizes an ancient and sacred yoga practice called "Mula Bandha" as a con-firmed method to treat and even *prevent* stress incontinence, or that spring-loaded sex toys have been clinically proven to strengthen the interior pubococcygeal (PC) muscle surrounding the urethra and control the flow of urine.

HAVE IT YOUR WAY

Youthful romps in the hay are typified by easy erections, volumi-nous lubrication, surefire penetrative sex, and explosive orgasms. As the decades roll by, this sequence frequently loses its sizzle. Reasons may vary. Perhaps you just aren't as "into it" as you used to be. Maybe his erections aren't as quick or hard. Perhaps your lovemaking routine has gone stale. Never you mind. It's high time you move past male-oriented, wham-bam-thank-you-ma'am sexual encounters anyway.

While women have been conditioned to regard lack of desire or any degree of sexual dysfunction as not-to-be-discussed disappoint-ments, I encourage you to throw back the covers and consider this: The time it takes you to get in the mood or for his equipment to get into gear can be all yours. Most women need about twenty min-utes of thinking about sex before their bodies are primed for full response. Now your precoitus warm-up can benefit you both. Ask for and receive all the snuggling, caressing, and oral sex you have craved for years and he'll have plenty of time to gladly oblige.

Consider the following tips to spark a fresh attitude toward friskiness:

Read a book or watch a video on tantric sex. The goal of tantric sex is not the big "O"; instead, the techniques are intended to prolong the sexual experience, increase sexual energy, and heighten the experience of intimacy with your partner. Some women report that by channeling the sexual energy that would normally leave their bodies during orgasm, they achieve a state akin to temporary enlightenment. According to Christiane Northrup, MD, author of *Women's Bodies, Women's Wisdom*, "Through the prolonged, intimate connection with another, women's nasty stress hormone levels lower while health- and life-enhancing oxytocin and serotonin levels shoot through the roof."

Turn it off with a flare. Look him in the eye, kiss him fully on the lips (tongue preferred), then pull back and put your finger on the off button of your cell phone. Next, walk your phone into another room and leave it. Return and reach for his. Repeat. Then undress as you walk back. Odds are he won't worry about the messages he might be missing.

Explore new regions. The base of your spine is erotica waiting, so turn over and let him touch and taste. Also ask him to gently stroke and kiss your belly just above the pubic hairline.

Go to new heights. Hike to the top of a fire tower, book a room on the twenty-fifth floor with a floor-to-ceiling window, or make out in a hot-air balloon. The point is, when you have little between the two of you but sky, your sense of limitation falls away. And that breathless feeling of being almost off the edge will heighten the urgency and excitement of every touch.

Have a mint. Place a jigger of peppermint schnapps or crème de menthe on your bedside table. Put your finger in the liquor, then in his mouth. Have him do the same with you. Then experiment with edible finger painting. The cool mint sensation plus breath and tongue on breasts and genitals guarantees a new kind of buzz.

Teach him the joyful game of start and stop. This is a tried-and-true method of helping men last longer in bed. Pay attention to when he's approaching his point of no return, then use body language (or ask) to change positions. He'll calm down a bit and most likely oblige you with a few more minutes of oral or manual stimulation until he is fully aroused again.

Trade report cards. So what if you can't get pregnant? You are never too old to contract sexually transmitted diseases (STDs). Recent statistics show a growing rate of STDs in the over-fifty crowd, even among the nursing home population. So, anytime you are sexually active with a new partner, don't be coy. Buy the condoms until he provides *current lab work* validating negative results for all STDs. And be fair—give him yours.

No Sex, No Worries:
You Are a Cocreative Powerhouse

I hate bugs, particularly roaches and swarming things that bite. Consequently, a mid-August trip to a home on the banks of North Florida's Ichetucknee River was a guaranteed descent into personal purgatory.

"Tell me again why you're going to see some old lady in the woods?" Randy asked.

"Kathleen told me this woman Dailey is an unbelievable artist who makes exquisite masks and figures out of dead animal bones. I'm interviewing her for my chapter on cocreation. You know, about how when you partner with the Divine, you can create new life even from things broken, decaying, or thought dead."

Randy rolled his eyes. "Sounds like modern-age voodoo, but whatever. If you're going to spend the night, you should take my pistol. What do you really know about this woman? Who knows what kind of weirdo she might be?"

Forgoing the pistol, I loaded up on insect repellant, pen, paper, and a tape recorder. After two and a half hours on isolated roads, I stopped to pee behind a bush. Didn't occur to me to fear snakes, and, for the moment, bugs were on hiatus, so I walked through dense trees down to the riverbank. A white-tailed doe raised her head to stare at me before returning to drink from crystalline water. Unnerved, I hurried back to my ordinary car, turned on National Public Radio, and determined to find Dailey's house before sunset.

Soon after, I pulled into a dirt driveway next to a petite red cabin nestled under oaks and pines. A note on the door read, "Ran out for wine. Be back in a jiff. Come on in."

I cracked the door and stood transfixed.

With light golden walls, a dusk blue ceiling, and sheer peach silk curtains, the last sunbeams through the windows transformed Dailey's studio into a veritable sunset. On the walls hung intricately jeweled, hand-painted animal skulls, as large as bison and as small as a cardinal. They, too, sent prisms of color across walls and floor. The fattest cat I had ever seen raised its head from a crimson pillow, blinked, then lowered back to sleep.

A rich chuckle broke my reverie. "I'm so glad you got here in time. Was afraid you would miss my nightly rainbow."

I turned to face a wiry woman with short gray hair and dancing eyes—one of the most enigmatic, sensual women I have ever encountered.

As with Dailey, art can be sensual outlet and expression for many women. Others express their innate sexuality through dance and movement. In fact, clinical data validates that women often go beyond intercourse to enliven their sexuality in a number of creative modalities.

A survey of more than eight hundred women between the ages of forty to one hundred found that almost half of the women surveyed had not had sex in a month, yet they declared themselves "sexually satisfied." On the surface, these findings in the January 2012 edition of the *American Journal of Medicine* appear contradictory, a conundrum. Then the fine print comes into focus.

The study's authors suggest that, for older women, the sexual experience moves far beyond literal intercourse. They suggest the experience of nurturing, affirming, and sustaining relationships become female-enlivened sexual activities. This new definition of sexuality embraces our ageless and ever-present creative power; in other words, our divinely derived, cocreative power.

Women are natural-born incubators and creators. In our reproductive years, our innate sexual vitality, plus copulating with a male, plus fertilization of the ovum (egg) can lead to children. This sequence, termed "procreation," works properly for a limited number of decades. Also, a man—or at least his sperm—is requisite.

On the other hand, sexual vitality, plus an openness to partner with your Higher Power, combined with inspired action unifies Spirit and matter. This "cocreative" phenomenon can occur at any age but, typically, becomes richer and deeper with age.

Sometimes a woman's cocreative energy becomes tangible via art, music, writing, gardening, leadership development, new business ventures, sports enthusiasm, or philanthropic passion. Other times, a more subtle, interior birthing occurs, one evidenced by deeper joy and greater serenity regarding life's inevitable beauty and brutality.

I was in my early thirties when my professional functioning in a male-dominated healthcare business environment had become flat, stale, and lackluster. A friend suggested I try something new to recharge my creative batteries: a drumming circle. The idea was way out of my comfort zone, but I decided to give it a roll. Intent on always being fashion-appropriate, I donned calf-high boots (in case of snakes or varmints), bought a flowered peasant dress from a vintage store, and put my hair in braids.

I arrived at a farmhouse on the outskirts of Nashville looking like a past-my-prime, wannabe flower child. Thankfully, the other women in pressed jeans and button-down shirts didn't comment. They simply opened their circle a little wider. Then a beautiful red-head named Suchi Waters Benjamin (who now lives in Maui and is the founder of the Center for Co-Creative Living) handed me a small drum and began to sing. My master's level training in neural processing, for example, using right-brain rhythms to reprogram linear left-brain thinking, immediately (and for the very first time) shifted from academic to personal.

Writing is something I never imagined doing or had any formal training in. Still, the sequence between inspiration and transcription merges my inborn feminine creativity with my more masculine inclination to get things done. Like a mother holding a newborn, I behold each word, page, and book a miracle. I fully believe *Fountain of Truth* was incepted two decades ago in my drumming circle on that Tennessee farm.

PART THREE

A FRESH LOOK AT ANTI-AGING TRUTHS AS OLD AS DIRT

FORTY-SOMETHING HOLLIS WILDER appears to effortlessly bridge superbeautiful, supersavvy and supermogul. A wife, mother of two, successful businesswoman, and owner of cupcake stores Sweet! by Holly, Hollis is best known as two-time winner of *Cupcake Wars* and star of the Cooking Channel. She has also written a sure-to-be-bestseller cookbook, *Savory Bites: Meals You Can Make in Your Cupcake Pan.* Talk about a paradigm shifter: cupcake pans as our template for healthy portion control!

"Getting older is not easy but it's worth it. I like myself more every decade, and I'm told I look better and better with time," Hollis said firmly. "I attribute my positive aging to three things. The first is that I am clear on the fact that I am a product, a consequence, of my choices. You know, the whole 'reap what you sow' philosophy. I clearly own the truth that who I am, who I become, is up to my attitude, my preparation, and my effort. My life continues to improve because I choose to be tenaciously positive regardless of setbacks or sad things that happen, and I work hard at the other stuff too . . . health and lifestyle choices upping my ante of being sharp, svelte, and super-fun at fifty, sixty, seventy, and beyond. The second is I have a tight group of girlfriends. They know me. They both have my back and call me on my crap. My girlfriends are my go-to lifeline. The third is I am honest about the squirrelly stuff."

"What does that mean?" I put my pen down and leaned in.

"Let's first clarify what it means to get better, not older. Enviable women have lives that, on most days, overflow with meaning, love, joy, and good health. I say 'most days' because we all have bad days, live on a flawed planet, and know sad things happen to good people. For the most part, however, women who feel and look great no matter their age experience life on the upswing. My experience is that women aging poorly have individual versions of sad, squirrelly little secrets. They constantly blame their less-than-optimum personal circumstance on others or bad luck. They play life out as victims. They whine. Women aging poorly might say they want a fit body and good health, but their actions tell another story. Maybe it's drinking too much or food bingeing. Maybe it's choosing mindless television over an hour of exercise. Maybe it's staying in a dysfunctional marriage. Maybe it's overspending. It doesn't matter. I am convinced that the lies we tell ourselves and act out every day accelerate our decay."

Hollis mirrored what I heard from hundreds of women aging in enviable fashion: We are the consequence of our individual choices and actions. This mind-set is psychologically termed a "strong internal locus of control." Conversely, people with an "external locus of control" believe the quality of their life depends on luck and other people. They are the whiners and victims.

STUFF HAPPENS

Live long enough and stuff happens. First, and sometimes second and third, loves fizzle. Career aspirations go flat, or there is downsizing at work. People we thought we could count on disappoint. Children get in trouble, break our hearts. Sometimes retirement funds blow away like a dandelion in the wind. You, or someone you love, gets really sick. Then there is death, as immutable as gravity but oh-so-much-more heartsickening when the loss is someone you love.

Women with a strong internal locus of control refuse to be buckled by stuff, including inevitable mistakes, disappointments, heartaches, and the physical marks of years passing by. They learn—and intrinsically grow more desirable, beautiful, and resilient—as a result. Women lacking a strong internal locus of control tend to squander precious time and energy grieving both what happened to them and what never did. Women lacking a strong internal locus of control also tend to use food as an emotional buffer.

FOOD FOR THOUGHT

Clare Lavendar, PhD, holistic nutritionist and dear friend, recently introduced me to the concept of primary foods versus secondary foods. The philosophy is the foods you eat are secondary to all the other things that feed you—your relationships, career, spirituality, and exercise routine. Those things are regarded as primary foods. Secondary foods are what you put into your mouth and swallow. The premise is, if your primary foods are in balance and satisfying, you won't crave foods that sabotage your waistline, your health, and how quickly you age.

I reached out to Nan Allison, MS, RD, LDN, coauthor with Carol Beck of *Full and Fulfilled: The Science of Eating to Your Soul's Satisfaction.* Nan's ongoing clinical work and research examines why we choose to eat the way we do. She explained: "Most people, and particularly women, use food to celebrate, comfort, nurture, distract, and numb out. Anxiety, loneliness, boredom, and anger all send triggers to our brain that associate with eating. Most women then use food like a drug in an effort to quell their core feelings. Some women do the reverse. They don't eat, literally attempting to starve their feelings away."

According to Evelyn Tribole, MS, RD, and Elyse Resch, MS, RD, FADA, authors of *Intuitive Eating*, "Food won't solve the problem. If anything, eating for an emotional hunger will only make you feel worse in the long run. You'll ultimately have to deal with the source of the emotion, as well as the discomfort of overeating."

What You Need Now

A strong internal locus of control is not for purchase, and no one can give it to you. It is a deeply ingrained thinking pattern that typically starts early in life and then develops over a period of years, but it's never too late to learn how to think differently. No matter how old or young you are, you can start right now to build your internal locus of control muscles. The following will help:

- Faith in a Higher Power
- A good group of girlfriends
- A commitment to laugh often and play more
- Taking up a sport
- A good marriage
- A purpose to give back now and leave a legacy once gone.

CHAPTER 10

FAITH—A PROVEN PATH TO WELLNESS

I N MY TWENTIES AND THIRTIES I WAS AN overachieving, stressed-to-the-max, whirling-dervish workaholic. My astonishing evolution into a more calm, joyful, and purposeful person began accidentally. On a lark with a girlfriend, I found myself naked in a hot tub overlooking Big Sur, conversing with an elder Benedictine monk (Brother David Steindl-Rast) about the meaning of my life.

Don't spritz your knickers thinking I am going to tell you that to decelerate your aging, you too have to go cross-country and get into a hot tub with a monk. As we get older, there is less need for extreme drama; moreover, active faith does not require a kickoff event. Millions of women of faith confirm that an ingrained and intentional belief in a Higher Power works best when quietly radiating through each moment of every day.

Like the mystical Sufis, I personally believe there are as many paths to God as there are breaths of children. Accordingly, when I speak of a Higher Power, I am not endorsing a specific religiosity. Whatever name you call your God or Higher Power, I am rallying you to press into your faith.

I have grown very intentional about nurturing my faith. I start every morning with a "coffee with God" hour. I pray, journal, and read my devotionals. I also surround myself with Spirit-enlivened women.

Phyllis Tousey is right down the road, reading her Bible as the sun rises over the Atlantic Ocean. I can close my eyes and feel the sparks from Debbie Austin's prayers igniting her ministry. Rhonda Marko tells me she prays aloud in her car. With the advent of Blue-tooth technology, people pulling alongside think she is talking on the phone. Stacey Graham shares an inspirational quote on her voice-mail message. Passing time during chemo treatments, Linda Cunningham texts me daily meditation messages. Marjean Coddon nudges me to bridge from my Christian heritage to also embrace the wisdom of the Kabbalah. Sue Fort White and I both read *Daily Word* and *God Calling*. I know if I call her at any time to ask advice, we'll begin our conversation from the same spiritual context.

Consider the following: spiritually active women are healthier, have longer life expectancies, and experience enhanced quality of living.

THE SCIENCE OF SPIRITUALITY

Ascending the steps of the red-brick, white-columned house of eighty-five-year-old Velma Morris, I cursed the airline that lost my bag. Mrs. Morris was the South's first recognized female religious writer. It had taken me more than three years to finagle an interview. Now, sans black suit with pearls, I would be on her doorstep wearing none-too-clean stretch jeans, an old sweatshirt, and a thirty-year-old pair of clogs (yes, clogs; they slide off easy in the airport security line and keep my feet warm on the plane). So much for first impressions.

I knocked, expecting a maid to open the door, take one look, and shoo me off the premises. Instead Mrs. Morris greeted me in black sweats and a white apron, looking like a plump, blue-haired penguin. A stereo blaring Frankie Valli's "Big Girls Don't Cry" drowned out her greeting.

Over deviled eggs, celery stuffed with homemade pimento cheese, and ham sandwiches on oven-warm bread, we got down to business. Our conversation would leave an inestimable mark on me.

"Please don't call me a 'religious writer.' That label makes me feel like I am selling God as if he were a good used car. I simply write about everyday people asking the same questions humans have asked since the beginning of time: Why do men fight wars? Why do children get cancer and other terminal illnesses? Why are some people blessed with prosperity so stingy? Why haven't you caused the penis to drop off every man who participates in or condones female genital mutilation? What's really going to happen to me when I die?

"Honey, I'm a Christian and Reverend Morris was an ordained Presbyterian minister, but if he were alive he'd tell you the same thing I'm about to. The common denominator in the sacred texts of all faiths is this: Choosing to be at peace regardless of what's going on in your life or our world is feet-hit-the-street faith in

> Choosing to be at peace regardless of what's going on in your life or our world is feet-hit-the-street faith in action. In the daily battle between good and evil, sickness and health, it's our ultimate trump card.

action. In the daily battle between good and evil, sickness and health, it's our ultimate trump card."

Mayo Clinic backs up Mrs. Morris's premise. "Nurture your spirit no matter what you call your source of inspiration," a Mayo Clinic health letter advises, then cites research for credibility. Duke University studied four thousand people for four years and found that those who attended church weekly had a 28 percent lower mortality rate overall when compared to those who didn't belong to a church community. The researchers also considered income, education, chronic diseases, other illnesses, health habits, exercise, smoking, drinking, body fat, social participation, and psychological status. *None* of these factors explained the results.

Other research shows people who are regularly involved in religious and spiritual activities statistically live longer than those who are not. Church attendance was the strongest predictor of longevity. Various theories have been put forth to explain this spiritual dimension of longevity. Physical explanations include the fact that people who are involved in religious groups benefit from the social networks they form. If they get sick, others look out for them. Religious beliefs may also lead to less risky behavior.

In addition, a well-developed sense of spirituality may help people better cope with life's tough psychological demands. In a later study done by Duke University of 1,700 older Americans, researchers at Duke University Medical Center found that those who attend religious services had stronger immune responses. About 60 percent of the men and women surveyed attended religious services at least once a week. Blood tests showed that regular attendees were less likely to have a high level of an immune system protein involved in age-related diseases. This study suggests a direct positive effect.

PRAYER, MEDITATION, AND THE RELAXATION RESPONSE

Surveys indicate that nearly 90 percent of patients with serious illness will engage in prayer for the alleviation of their suffering or disease. Among all forms of complementary medicine, prayer is the single-most widely practiced healing modality. Prayer is the second-most common method of pain management (after oral pain medication) and the most common nondrug method of pain management.

A well-noted study by Dr. Herbert Benson, a cardiovascular medicine specialist at Harvard Medical School, documented the potential healing benefits of spiritual practices, such as prayer and meditation (as well as hypnosis and other relaxation techniques). Benson demonstrated that the body responds to these practices with what he calls the relaxation response, which consists of "a lowering of the heart rate, blood pressure, and breathing rate; a reduced need for oxygen; less carbon dioxide production." In effect, the relaxation response is the opposite of the stress response and can be consciously used to modulate the impact of stress.

Some of the effects of prayer may be due to the larger context within which prayer occurs, which is usually one of religious commitment and social support.

Medical researchers believe prayer improves health in the following ways:

The relaxation response: prayer elicits the relaxation response, which lowers blood pressure and other factors heightened by stress.

Secondary control: prayer releases control to something greater than oneself, which can reduce the stress of needing to be in charge.

The placebo response: prayer can enhance a person's hopes and expectations, and that in turn can positively impact health.

Healing presence: prayer can bring a sense of a spiritual or loving presence and alignment with God or an immersion into a universal unconsciousness.

Positive feelings: prayer can elicit feelings of gratitude, compassion, forgiveness, and hope, all of which are associated with healing and wellness.

Mind-body-spirit connection: when prayer uplifts or calms, it inhibits the release of cortisol and other hormones, thus reducing the negative impact of stress on the immune system and promoting healing.

FAITH IN ACTION

Dr. Pam Chally, dean of Brooks College of Health at the University of North Florida, and a beautiful blond with enviable skin and kickstart brain, shares: "My core belief is we are all here to serve. I grew up on a farm. My high school graduating class had only forty-six people in it. You might have thought my youth would give me a small view of the world. But, you see, faith was the fabric of both my family and my community. And faith has no bounds. Even as a little girl, I believed with God all things are possible. I continue to live that out today."

God is doing a lot with Dean Chally. She was awarded *Health-Source* magazine's 2012 Celebration of Nurses award and has received the EVE award for Education, UNF Distinguished Professor, Desmond Tutu Peace and Reconciliation Award, the Transformational Leadership and Collaborative Engagement Award, and was honored as a Woman of Influence by the *Jacksonville Business Journal*. Despite the hoopla, she contends, "My greatest accomplishment will always be to stay present, not get preoccupied, so I can treat everyone—whether the janitor or the president—with a high level of respect, love, and honor."

Carla Harris is a managing director in the Institutional Advisory Group at Morgan Stanley Investment Management. She is also the author of *Expect to Win* and a gospel singer who sells out Carnegie Hall. Carla has been on the following lists: *Fortune* magazine's "The Most Powerful Black Executives in Corporate America" and "The Most Influential List" (2005), *Black Enterprise* magazine's "Top 50 African Americans on Wall Street," *Essence* magazine's "The 50 Women Who Are Shaping the World," *Ebony* magazine's "15 Corporate Women at the Top," and the *Network Journal's* 2005 list of "25 Most Outstanding Women in Business." She was also named "Woman of the Year 2004" by the Harvard University Black Men's Forum. When it comes to how faith has shaped her aging, Carla says, "My faith is the center of my life; it is part of everything I do, including my business. My faith is what keeps me positive. I could say about aging, 'Oh, boy, I'm aging and things don't work the way they used to,' or I can say, 'One of the great benefits of aging is the cultivation of a discerning spirit. I get quiet for a few minutes, check in with prayer, and quickly know if I should be doing X versus Y. Now, in my fifties, I have a way of discerning things that was not possible in my twenties or thirties.'"

"Note: I believe there is a world of difference between wisdom and discernment. Wisdom evolves from my learning from the experiences God puts in my way. Discernment takes wisdom a step farther down a spiritual path. When I really don't know, don't have a clue what the right answer is, I can tune in and let God tell me what is right. You see, I would never have had the spiritual muscles for that much trust in my youth."

Listening to God saved Laura Bergman's (Laura B.) life. Laura B. shared how, in 2006, she resigned from the board of a large national philanthropy company, knowing that her best work was done there: "I wasn't sure what was next, but I felt a pregnant sense of purpose. I prayed and prayed and would get guidance like 'clean out your closets,' 'straighten out yours and Tom's personal accounting record,' and 'fix up your home a bit.' It was tempting to be frustrated because I had this sense that my purpose was bigger, but I disciplined myself to obey. Better to follow God's nudges with a cheerful heart. This went on for a year."

"Then, in April 2007, after a routine mammogram, I was told there was a suspicious area in my breast that could 'possibly one day, maybe, turn into breast cancer.' I prayed for guidance and God told me to go for a second opinion. I did immediately and soon learned I definitely had breast cancer not in one, but both, breasts. If I hadn't prayed, listened, and acted on Divine Guidance, who knows if I would be alive today."

TALKING ABOUT TRUSTING YOUR INSTINCTS

Laura B. shared how, immediately upon her diagnosis, she asked a question. The answer to her question would lay out God's purpose for the next several years of her life: "I said 'I would like to speak to a woman who has the exact kind of breast cancer I have so she can tell me from her own experience what I might expect.' The doctors at Mayo told me they didn't have any kind of patient-to-patient sharing system. I knew right then and there the mission God had been preparing me for: to start a breast cancer advocacy program. I couldn't have done it, or done it with peace of mind, if I hadn't spent the year before getting my house in order."

Laura B. is founder of Pink Sisters and Friends advocacy group at Mayo Clinic in Florida. The program serves hundreds of women each year, matching the diagnosis and protocol of each new breast cancer patient with a Pink Sister advocate with the same. The two women stay together, in constant contact, throughout treatment. Together they tackle the gritty stuff: doctor and hospital appointments, dealing with surgeries, chemotherapy, radiation and its effects, and home care after surgery, as well as psychological, familial, financial, and sexual challenges. Laura B. has been nominated for the L'Oréal Paris 2012 Women of Worth Award, which recognizes and honors women making an exceptional difference in their communities.

UNBELIEF ON THE UPTICK

According to a 2012 report from the Pew Center, the number of people in the United States who say they believe in "nothing in particular" is on the rise. Barry Kosmin, coauthor of three American Religious Identification Surveys, theorizes why "None" has become the "default category." He says, "Young people are resistant to the authority of institutional religion, older people are turned off by the politicization of religion, and people are simply less into theology than ever before."

Kosmin's surveys were the first to brand the "Nones" in 1990 when they were 6 percent of US adults. By the 2008 survey, "Nones" were up to 15 percent. By 2010, another survey, the biannual General Social Survey, bumped the number to 18 percent.

Ladies, I am not here to evangelize, but these statistics raise grave concerns. If faith in a Higher Power is the single most defining variable of our aging and quality of life, then even a slight trend in growing disbelief is an insidious risk factor. It raises the bar for all women of faith: Are you—am I—living a life that other women and girls want to emulate? Do you and I look, act, and smile like we have something they should want?

CHAPTER 11

GIRLFRIENDS ARE NEXT TO GOD

A T FORTY-TWO, I MET AN OLDER WOMAN who became
my friend and, through her love and counsel, filled in many
of the blank spaces my mother left behind. She would also open the
door to new directions for my life

It was 2002 and I was worn out from a corporate turnaround, so I
decided to take a sabbatical. I leased my house in Nashville, packed
up Bodhisattva (Bodhi, my shih tzu), Namaste (Nami, my marma-
lade-colored kitty), several pairs of cutoffs, and my computer to head
to Apalachicola, a tiny town in Florida's panhandle. My girlfriends
thought I was crazy.

"It doesn't have a traffic light. You're kidding, right?"

"Does FedEx even deliver there?"

"The grocery store is called the what? The Piggly Wiggly?"

"I've been there. It's pretty, but you know there are no single men, at least none who still have their own teeth."

But I was undeterred, fixated. Today I look back and wonder why. I can only conclude it was a God thing.

My move wasn't seamless. I fractured my foot and the moving truck went missing for three days. Geoff, one of my new neighbors, knocked on the door of the house I had rented to warn, "You know, gators are right out there in the bay at the end of your yard. They're likely to think that puppy and kitty of yours are fancy hors d'oeuvres."

Yikes! For the first time I wondered if I might have made a huge mistake.

My third day I woke at dawn and watched the sunrise over the bay. I remember feeling exquisitely peaceful, then jumping up, panicking. Nami wasn't on my bed. Or in the house. I threw on a pair of cutoffs, put on my protective boot, pulled my hair into a ponytail, and hobbled out in search.

I called and called. No Nami. I looked all over my yard, even tiptoeing down to the edge of the bay. No Nami. I could hear Bodhi frantically barking in the house. I started crying. Then I saw her, all five pounds of yellow fur, scampering into a hedge in the yard next door. I hadn't yet met this neighbor, but I had been told she was an older woman whose husband was in the nursing home—and also that she had a very sophisticated security system. Seeing a light in the window, I decided best to knock on the door and announce myself before foraging for Nami in her bushes.

I knocked. The door opened.

"Hi, I'm Genie James and I just moved next door. I am sorry to bother you so early, but my cat is hiding in your hedge. I need to catch her and take her home, but I didn't want you to be scared if you looked out your window and saw a strange woman in a boot going through your bushes."

Twinkling eyes looked me up and down. The woman pursed her lips for a second then seemed to relax. She smiled.

"Do you play bridge, honey? Our fourth died last week."

"No, ma'am. I am sorry, but I don't."

"Oh well. Do you drink wine?"

"Yes, ma'am, I do."

She brightened. "Now that's nice. I'll see you over here this afternoon at five."

With that, Smiles Randolph, my new best friend, Randy's mother, and my future mother-in-law, closed her door.

THE HORMONE CONNECTION

Clinical studies show girlfriends give more than psychological and emotional benefit. A cohort of supportive women can have a positive impact on the immune system, cardiac and breast health, pain response, and even reduce the chances of catching a cold. According to UCLA researchers Drs. Laura Klein and Shelley Taylor, bonding with women stimulates the release of a hormone called "oxytocin," which has a calming, peaceful effect. The positive effects of oxytocin are enhanced by the presence of estrogen, which circulates in the system of even non-menstruating women. This calming response doesn't happen in men because testosterone, the male dominant hormone, blocks oxytocin's positive neurological stimulation.

Girlfriends Shore Up
Inner Locus of Control

I am certain that if it were not for my girlfriends and my sister Sheila, I would be either loony or dead. They help me through life's rough patches, celebrate my successes, and nudge (or pull) me into a better future. Most of all, my girlfriends hold me accountable for my choices.

Stacey was with me the last time I saw Mother alive and the first time I dared tell a large audience stories from my heart. Pat has helped me negotiate multiple life contracts, from business to personal, ensuring I hang on to what's my due and come out ahead. Suebee was the first to nudge me down an authentic spiritual path and continues to counsel my sometimes knee-jerk personality to "pray, listen, wait, then act."

Shirley bailed me out of a jam, then helped me get a job. Aleene proves that those you love in junior high can sometimes grow up and old with you. She and Fran are strong threads weaving back into my memory what was good from our childhood. Kay shows me by example how our God is a God of second and third new beginnings.

Vicki never judges when I land in deep doo-doo. She cheerfully shows up with a shovel and helps me get a plan. Marjean always listens, then creates a safe place for me to be scared before I can be strong. By juggling sickness, a business, and single motherhood, Linda teaches me how courage, tenacity, and tenderness never go out of style.

GIRLFRIENDS CAN BE A LIFELINE

I saw Linda yesterday. Only a week and she looked at least ten pounds thinner, weight she didn't have to lose. And she was befuddled. I've seen it before, too many times: chemo brain. I feel angry: Why her? Helpless: What can I do? My homemade four-cheese macaroni casserole won't help.

Linda has chutzpah, tenacity, and a tight girlfriend group who have known her and loved her actively for decades. I'm new to this sisterhood. Though they might be wary of a stranger in their midst, these women understand Linda is going to need all the help she can get. So they include me. We'll show up, do what—no *all*—we can. Thankfully, Linda's long-term prognosis is excellent. Still, Smiles and Laura taught me the hardest life lesson: No matter how much we pray, love and give of ourselves we can't cancel out sickness. Or cheat death when it's time. But girlfriends can sometimes tip the balance back in our favor. Consider Maggie's story:

> In November of 1998 I was diagnosed with late-stage ovarian cancer —stage 3-C—which is one step away from stage 4 (e.g., worst-case scenario). The cancer hadn't yet spread to my lungs, but it had spread to other parts of my body. I was forty-five, recently widowed (my husband had been killed the year before in a car accident), and the mother of seven-year-old twin boys.
>
> My gynecologist told me there were factors in my favor: my relatively young age and the fact that I was fit and had never smoked. Still, the first oncologist said I had only a 20 to 30 percent chance of being alive in five years. For seconds I sat stunned; then I stood up.
>
> "Your statistics will not define my future," I said, walking out his door.
>
> I got into my parked car and cried, then started calling and calling.

My girlfriends. There are twelve of us who have loved each other since junior high. All were at my home the following evening, three flying cross-country to show up.

We made a pact. I would choose to live. And if/when I wanted to give up, my girlfriends would take turns standing by my side and whispering in my ear until I was strong enough to once again choose life.

That first year was the hardest. For starters I underwent something called "debulking" surgery. The surgeon was able to get only 75 percent of the cancer out. Then I suffered through six months of aggressive chemotherapy. Never a day went by that I didn't hear from all eleven girlfriends. One or two were always with me, holding my head over the toilet or doing the day-to-day chores of mothering my boys.

When I missed midget football games, one girlfriend videotaped them. Another sewed a flannel nightgown in school colors, making me a legitimate bed-bound cheerleader. Delicious breakfasts, lunches, and dinners appeared like room service. Weekly movie night became a new tradition. Requisite: only movies with very happy endings.

When I lost my hair, eyebrows, and lashes, we took over the wig salon, poured champagne, and determined I shun sandy brown locks for flamboyant, curly tresses. Orange, I was told, radiates warmth and energy while stimulating appetite, activity, and socialization. My demure, no-frills self somersaulted. "Orange curly hair? Why not?"

My new oncologist enrolled me in a study following fifty women with advanced ovarian cancer. The study was designed to evaluate correlation between social support—or lack thereof—and levels of an inflammatory protein called interleukin-6, or IL-6. High levels of IL-6 are linked to a poorer prognosis for women with ovarian cancer.

Every three months for the first year and every six months for the past eleven, I have sat down with a psychologist. Absent a husband or lover, I am cynically probed as to how "only girlfriends" could adequately meet innate needs for closeness, intimacy, and nurturance. Despite multiple interviewers' skepticism, I unfailingly score highest in social support. Other numbers illuminate my scores' significance: that first year my IL-6 scores were consistently 70 percent lower than my peers. Remember: the lower, the better. Even better, my lower than average IL-6 scores have remained stable for more than a decade. The most bittersweet number: of the original fifty women in the study, I am the only one remaining.

LOCUS OF CONTROL MAKES A FRIEND, FINDS HOPE, AND A FUTURE

"It is because of Kristi that I am here, well and working. Kristi also helped my whole family have a better life," said Habiba.

Habiba, a Bosnian immigrant, first came to the United States after suffering heinous atrocities during her country's civil war. Through near-starvation, untreated illness, untended pregnancy, barbaric living conditions, not knowing if her young husband was dead or alive, and being separated from her infant daughter, Habiba says she never considered giving up.

"It is hard to describe the kind of fear that lived in my heart, but I never forgot that I had to do everything I could to stay strong, to be positive. I had to look forward."

Obviously, this woman has an internal locus of control to envy, but what exactly was it that Habiba looked forward to?

In 1999, reunited with her husband and daughter, Habiba came to the United States. Though educated, she spoke little English, so she got the only job she could, working for an office building cleaning service in Jacksonville, Florida. One night while emptying a trash can, she met Kristi.

"When I met Kristi I was already very sick," Habiba shared, "but I tried not to focus on that. Instead, I would come into this important woman's office in the early evening and try to be quiet so as to not disturb her work. But she talked to me. She asked me questions about my life and my family. She genuinely seemed to care."

Habiba, only in her late twenties, was experiencing painful joint symptoms. She was soon diagnosed with rheumatoid arthritis and told by her doctor that, unless she began aggressive therapy immediately, she would be in a wheelchair before age forty. But the treatment was expensive and she had no insurance.

"I could not allow myself to focus on that bad news," Habiba told me, "so I would spend hours before work prying my fingers open and massaging my hands and feet. Every movement became painful, even driving. Still, I believed God would not have helped me survive the war unless I was needed to live to be a strong and good mother for my beautiful daughter. My choice was to give up, stay home and die, or keep showing up. I chose to show up. One thing that helped was that almost every night I worked, I would see Kristi."

"Kristi" is a petite blond daughter of a Baptist minister. She is also president of a Jacksonville Citibank site and a state officer for Florida, responsible for community and government relations, site work environment, and the overall culture of more than 4,800 employees. I asked about her hand in Habiba's life.

"I watched Habiba clean my office with more than meticulous dedication; she exuded something akin to reverence. I was struck by the way this warmly friendly yet surprisingly dignified young woman would quietly pick up and dust every one of my family pictures, particularly those of my son. I noticed she would look at those closely. I would learn my son is the same age as her daughter."

Despite language and barriers of class and station, Kristi and Habiba became friends. Their bond bore fruit. In 2002 Habiba became a Citibank employee. Today she works in the Quality Department for Transaction Services, where she was awarded a 2012 Quality Excellence Award because, during her entire tenure, she has made zero errors processing credit cards and serving customers.

Habiba's resilient internal locus of control is awe-inspiring. Nevertheless, it is Kristi's story I find most life-impacting. I ask myself, *Would I even have noticed Habiba emptying my trash can? Would I have bridged our differences to begin and sustain a conversation, much less foster a friendship? Would I have taken the risk of championing to my superiors the hiring of a cleaning woman with broken English and health issues?*

The old me would have said, "Probably not." Because of Habiba and Kristi's story, however, I would like to believe my answer today might very possibly be "Yes."

CHAPTER 12

LIGHTEN UP AND
PLAY MORE

PICTURE TWO TABLES OF WOMEN EATING LUNCH. At the
first table sit two friends smiling, laughing, and sharing an appe-
tizer. At the second table sit two scowling women robotically inhal-
ing their salads while checking text messages. At which table are the
women radiating health and well-being? Now, be honest. At which
table would you likely be sitting?

UNPLUG AND CHILL OUT

Forty-two year-old Velma knows she shouldn't text while driving,
so she compromises, putting her thumbs to work only at stop lights
or during traffic jams. Today a blaring horn and middle-finger-out-
the-window tells her she missed her light. Guiltily, Velma pockets
the phone in her purse.

She comes home, slips off her pantsuit, puts on sweats, and looks at the elliptical in the den off their bedroom. She has about an hour before Connor shows up with the kids. They had agreed to take turns carpooling to soccer practice to trade off an hour for working out every other night. Velma looks at the elliptical again and considers her increasingly smushy thighs. Then she plops on the bed, pulls her phone out of her purse, and begins checking e-mails. She's just logged onto Facebook when she hears Connor's car. Quickly, she stashes the phone, throws water on her face, and grabs a towel—just as she would have had she been working up a sweat.

"Web-based technology is no longer a convenience; it's my cocaine. My urge to log on is more irresistible than taking care of myself, spending time with my children, or having sex with Connor. Worse, I feel constantly anxious when unplugged."

Unfortunately, our multitasking, information-overloaded, instant-results-driven "Information Generation" is increasingly at risk of being chronically harried and exhausted as stalking to-do lists evoke gnawing guilt and growing feelings of inferiority. New research indicates heavy Internet use leads to something termed "popcorn brain," a condition where your brain becomes so accustomed to the constant stimulation of electronic multitasking that you become uncomfortable and unfit for life offline. Worse, other studies show insistent information fatigue can have harmful cognitive impact, leading women to use poorer judgment and make life-impacting choices they quickly regret.

Dr. Nora Volkow, director of the National Institute on Drug Abuse, explains that constant stimulation can activate dopamine cells in the nucleus accumbens, a main pleasure center of the brain. This simulates the addictive pleasure-seeking compulsion to never unplug. The looming doom is that over time, and with enough Internet usage, the structure of our brains can actually physically change.

Researchers in China did MRIs on the brains of eighteen college students who spent about ten hours a day online. Compared with a control group who spent less than two hours a day online, these students had less gray matter, the thinking part of the brain. A 2012 *Newsweek* review of findings from more than a dozen other countries showed similar trends.

While it may seem counterintuitive, one of the best health and beauty tips for any age is to chill out more. At a minimum, learn how to be "unavailable" for at least ten minutes three times a day. Get out of your house or office, or go to a room where you won't be disturbed. Leave your phone; at the very least, turn it off completely. Get practical to become unavailable.

I advise overbusy, high-demand women to do their best to chill out more. If nothing else, spend more time in the bathroom and take more showers, places you are less likely to be interrupted. Block out all noise and distractions, center yourself, discern between what you have the power to impact and what you do not, and cultivate calm.

LAUGHTER IS GOOD MEDICINE

Laughing is a neurotransmitter aphrodisiac. It also has an ecstatic ripple effect. According to my friend and "joyologist" Kathleen Halperin, "We've long known that the ability to laugh is helpful to those coping with major illness and the stress of life's problems. But researchers are now saying laughter can do a lot more—it can basically bring balance to all the components of the immune system, which helps us fight off diseases.

"Laughter provides a safety valve that shuts off the flow of stress hormones and the fight-or-flight compounds that swing into action in our bodies when we experience stress, anger, or hostility. These stress hormones suppress the immune system, increase the number of blood platelets (which can cause obstructions in arteries), and raise blood pressure.

"When we're laughing, natural killer cells that destroy tumors and viruses increase, as do gamma interferon (a disease-fighting protein), T cells (which are a major part of the immune response), and B cells (which make disease-destroying antibodies).

"Laughter may lead to hiccupping and coughing, which clears the respiratory tract by dislodging mucous plugs. Laughter also increases the concentration of salivary immunoglobulin A, which defends against infectious organisms entering through the respiratory tract.

"What may surprise you even more is the fact that researchers estimate that laughing one hundred times is equal to ten minutes on the rowing machine or fifteen minutes on an exercise bike. Laughing can be a total body workout! Blood pressure is lowered, and there is an increase in vascular blood flow and in oxygenation of the blood, which further assists healing. Laughter also gives your diaphragm and abdominal, respiratory, facial, and leg and back muscles a workout. That's why you often feel exhausted after a long bout of laughter—you've just had an aerobic workout!"

The psychological benefits of humor are quite amazing, according to doctors and nurses who are members of the American Association for Therapeutic Humor. People often store negative emotions, such as anger, sadness, and fear, rather than expressing them. Laughter provides a way for these emotions to be harmlessly released.

Laughter can also be cathartic. That's why some people who are upset or stressed out go to a funny movie or a comedy club, so they can laugh the negative emotions away (these negative emotions, when held inside, can cause biochemical changes that can affect our bodies). Increasingly, mental health professionals are suggesting "laughter therapy," which teaches people how to laugh—openly—at things that aren't usually funny and to cope in difficult situations by using humor.

LAUGH AT YOURSELF

The ability to laugh at ourselves allows us the opportunity to embrace our flaws and promotes self-acceptance. It does not include harmful put-downs, ridicule, or negative sarcasm. Nor are we advertising that we are defective; rather, we are demonstrating that we are human.

Humor is a positive coping mechanism that not only improves our mood, it builds our self-esteem. Unfortunately, we often resort to all kinds of unhealthy coping mechanisms like drinking, smoking, eating, overworking, and so on to make ourselves feel good. While these habits offer temporary boosts, they further undermine our self-esteem. Choose to laugh instead!

Tips for Laughing More Every Day

Watch a funny TV show every day (old syndicated sitcoms
are a great source of reliable laughs).

Read the daily comics online or in the newspaper.

Learn an age-appropriate joke and tell it to a youngster.
Making children laugh is one of the best ways to bring
more joy and humor into your life.

Subscribe to a joke, quip, or quote of the day and have the
laughs delivered right to your in-box.

Share funny articles with friends and family members.
Sometimes the thought of making someone else laugh
can give us the same sense of well-being we get when we
laugh at a joke. Reaching out to others with humor is a
wonderful way to strengthen connections and emotional
intimacy.

The Cheeky Science of Play

In March of 2012, my friend Pat Shea and I journeyed to Sante
Fe to attend a workshop on transformational speaking led by Gail
Larsen. The stated objective of the workshop was to help attendees
discover their "original medicine," for example, our singular gifts
and talents that define our unique, individual roles in influencing
change. I was skeptical that I had an original medicine, believing
my best talent was regurgitating helpful information and other people's good ideas. Regurgitate is synonymous with vomit. "Vomiter of
Other People's Stuff" didn't strike me as an original medicine name
people would gravitate toward.

Gail paired me with twenty-something Alexandra Franzen, who sported several mesmerizing tattoos and surprisingly red hair. Alexandra introduced herself: "I am half Jewish, half Swedish, a former lesbian, a recovering socialist, and a onetime helicopter pilot. I've moved through my strumpet years and my cubicle season to most recently establish myself as a quite successful entrepreneur."

Really? Partnering with this nascent, maverick beauty was supposed to help me become a better speaker and more intentional agent of change?

I looked at Gail. Raised my eyebrows. She smiled and nodded, pleased how well the two of us were bonding.

"Do you prefer Alex to Alexandra?"

"Only if you think you don't have time to say my whole name."

Oh boy. Fumbling for common ground, I asked "Alexandra" about her entrepreneurial business.

"Mostly, I play with words. In fact, *play* is my work."

Whoosh went my comfort zone. For the next five days Alexandra turned my thinking inside-out, explaining why playing every day is as critical to health, productivity, and creativity as sleep or food. Alexandra would later put her thinking to paper in her adorable book *50 Ways to Say You're Awesome* published by Sourcebooks, spring 2013.

Neurological science backs up Alexandra's premise. Our brains are made up of billions of neurons with connections between them. These neurons are bundled into groups called neural pathways. We have neural pathways for memory, attachment, emotions, language, motor control, each of our senses, and many more. When children and adults play, many parts of the brain are activated at the same time.

The brain "lights up" during a child's dramatic play: fine motor, gross motor, language, emotion, and memory; abstract concepts like "good guys" and "bad guys"; scientific concepts like cause and effect; social concepts like "taking care of baby"; and big themes like aggression, affection, loyalty, and power—each with its own neural pathway—are all seen during children's play.

Gary Landreth, professor at the University of North Texas, states that children act out their life experiences and feelings in a natural, dynamic, and self-healing manner. Play is the symbolic language children use for self-expression. When adults play, we begin to feel more positive because of a release of endorphins, and our stress levels go down. It calms and relaxes us while stimulating our brains and bodies. It helps us connect with others and increases our energy level and excitement. It is the antidote for loneliness, isolation, anxiety, and depression. It helps us feel happy, creative, and resilient.

Play is also the single best way for adults to simultaneously activate multiple neural pathways. If you want to know more, there is an Institute of Play and multiple books on the subject. My new fave is Stuart Brown's *Play: How It Shapes the Brain, Opens the Imagination, and Invigorates the Soul*. If, like me, you are hardwired to be a workaholic on overdrive, you also need to know:

Play has been scientifically proven to be good for the brain. All animals play. Grizzly bears that play the most survive the longest. Rats that socialize develop bigger, more complex brains. Play stimulates nerve growth in the portions of the brain that process emotions and executive function.

Play teaches us to use our imaginations. Imagination is perhaps the most powerful human ability, letting us create simulated realities we can explore without abandoning the real world. As kids grow older, the line between pretend and real becomes more solid, but imaginative play continues to nourish the spirit.

Rough-and-tumble play teaches us how to cooperate and play fair. Research in humans and animals has shown that roughhousing is necessary for the development of social awareness, cooperation, fairness, and altruism. If young rats are denied rough-and-tumble play, they develop serious social problems in adulthood and aren't able to mate.

Play helps us learn to be friends. When children are four to six years old, they start "mutual play," listening to other kids' points of view and incorporating them into imaginative games. This mutual play is the basic state of friendship that sustains us throughout our lives.

Sometimes the best way to learn a complicated subject is to play with it. That's why kids often learn computer systems faster than adults; they aren't afraid to just try stuff out and see what works. Kids don't fear doing something wrong. If they do, they learn from it and do it differently the next time.

Physical play delays mental decline in old age. Research on this is still in the early stages, but older people who get regular exercise are less likely to suffer cognitive decline. Doing crossword puzzles, brainteasers, and other thinking games seems to help, too.

A little play can help solve big problems. Play is nature's great tool for creating new neural networks and for reconciling cognitive difficulties. When we play, dilemmas and challenges naturally filter through the unconscious mind and work themselves out. Even a few hours spent doing something you love can make you new again.

When we get play right, all areas of our lives go better. One of the hardest things to teach kids is how to make it past difficulty or boredom to find the fun. Making all of life an act of play occurs when we recognize and accept that there may be some discomfort in play, and that every experience has both pleasure and pain.

My friend Alexandra has a black belt in play. Her work is her play and her play is her work, consequently, she has a hard time telling the difference between the two. I am still learning, but I do know this: Play means more than unplugging. It means freeing your mind to have fun. If you have forgotten how to play, borrow a three-year-old. Get on the floor or go outside. Let them reteach you. Even better, consider taking up a sport.

CHAPTER 13

PLAY MORE SPORTS

E LIZABETH NYE, DIRECTOR OF GIRLS, INC., in northwest Oregon, and I were on the phone. She said, "My life, my aging experience, is nothing like my grandmother's or my mother's. My grandmother grew up on a farm and never finished high school. In her adult years, she got up at four in the morning and walked to the nursing home where she worked as a kitchen aide. My mother got her high school diploma, married, worked as a secretary, and smoked her entire life. Relentless economic insecurity wore them down. Both were determined to create a different reality for me."

Boy, did they.

A graduate of Georgetown University's School of Foreign Service, Elizabeth started her career at Population Services International (PSI) in Washington, DC. While there, she worked on a variety of social marketing projects for malaria prevention, clean water, and HIV/AIDS prevention in the developing world. She then devoted the next five years to the pharmaceutical industry at Bristol-Myers

Squibb. As product manager in the company's Virology Division, she marketed HIV/AIDS products in the United States. She was also responsible for leading the Virology Division's Women's Initiative and African American Initiative to better understand and address the impact of HIV/AIDS on these populations. In 2006, Elizabeth relocated to her hometown of Portland, Oregon, with her husband and two daughters.

"So, when you think of the circumstances and perspectives associated with how you grew up compared to those surrounding your daughters today, what do you believe will be the most significant game changer?" I asked Elizabeth.

I assumed one of two responses to my question: education or more financial security. She surprised me by saying, "Sports. I think the fact that both my daughters are actively involved in sports teams will make the biggest difference."

Though I fully understood that playing a sport is a calorie-burning exercise with great social dynamics, it took me a while to buy into the power of sports as a vehicle for positive aging. Reflect back that I was the puny, asthmatic child kept indoors. When I did go to physical education, no one *ever* chose me to be on their kickball team. Not only was I sickly, I was—and continue to be—comically uncoordinated. I rang Donna Orender.

Donna, who lives near me in Jacksonville Beach, Florida, is a game changer of national scope. From 2003 to 2010 she served as president of the Women's National Basketball Association (WNBA). In 2005, Donna was named one of the ten most powerful women in sports by FOXSports.com.

"The data is undeniable. According to a survey of executive women, 81 percent played sports growing up and 69 percent said sports helped them to develop leadership skills contributing to their professional success." Many other women echoed Elizabeth's and Donna's thinking: "I believe my basketball experience can be directly linked to my business experience and success," said Mary Claire Bonner, who retired in 2009 from Aetna. Before retiring, the New York resident was senior vice president of local and regional business for Aetna, working directly for the company's president and "running a large business that concentrated on small and midsize employer health benefit needs in more than thirty states." Reflecting on the position, Bonner discovered that her favorite part about leading others was creating a strong team. The skills to be good at this, Bonner noted, started in fifth grade when she joined the basketball team.

"Playing basketball changed me as a person," said Bonner, who played from grade school through her junior year at one of Penn State's Commonwealth campuses.

According to the *Hall of Fame Network* magazine, the Women's Sports Foundation (started by female tennis champion Billie Jean King) became established because, "In an economic environment where the quality of our life is dependent on two-income families, our daughters cannot be less prepared for the highly competitive workplace than our sons."

Digging into the data, I was astounded by the correlation between sports and success among women, especially high-profile leaders. The key contributor was Title IX, a landmark legislation that celebrated its fortieth anniversary this year. A 2010 study by Betsey Stevenson, chief economist of the US Department of Labor, found that Title IX accounted for a 20 percent increase in women's education and for about a 40 percent rise in employment for women ages twenty-five to thirty-four.

In a 2012 column for CNN Money, Sanyin Siang, executive director of the Coach K Leadership and Ethics Center at Duke University, wrote, "Well documented are IMF managing director Christine Lagarde competing in synchronized swimming; PepsiCo CEO Indra Nooyi playing cricket; Kraft Foods CEO Irene Rosenfeld engaging in four varsity sports in high school and basketball in college; and HP CEO Meg Whitman playing lacrosse and squash.

"This is not surprising considering the mental discipline and social skills honed through playing sports. At the Coach K Center, we hear often from leaders such as Fidelity President Kathy Murphy, Walmart EVP of People Division Susan Chambers, and Morgan Stanley Managing Director Carla Harris about how sports had fostered the resilience, agility, and team-orientation that advanced their leadership. Also, engaging in and appreciating sports gives women an understanding of business parlance that is often steeped in sports analogies and provides another avenue for social inclusion in the workplace."

A Platform for Social Change

In the 2012 Summer Olympics, for the very first time, women athletes from Saudi Arabia were represented, and the US Olympic team had more women delegates than men. Women also made up 40 percent of the total number of athletes at the 2012 games.

In June 2012, Hillary Clinton announced the Global Sports Mentoring Program, saying, "We want to find ways to get more women and girls on the field, the court, the track, in the pool, the mat, wherever their interests and talents take them so they can discover their strengths, develop their skills, experience that special satisfaction that sports can bring, win or lose. And we believe in the positive effects that can flow out of that experience with girls and women across their lifetimes and, by extension, for their families and communities."

The 1984 Olympic gold medalist Nawal El Moutawakel says, "Sport is one of the best tools for social change because it is a large part of cultures around the world and reaches into every socioeconomic class of society. Sport helps develop self-esteem and confidence, improve physical and mental well-being, serve as a medium of communication, and empower women to improve themselves and their communities."

I called my niece Shelley and asked her to chime in. Shelley is director of development for Explore Austin, a six-year committed mentoring program for underserved girls and boys. Think leadership development meets Outward Bound–type vision quests, including strenuous hiking and rock climbing to get a sense of Explore Austin's model: "What we have seen with our youth in these programs is that moving through the realms of physical exertion, collaboration, and teamwork creates deep bonds of trust difficult to ignite through only conversation. Taking young women out of their comfort range to stretch them physically, mentally, and emotionally is a dynamic engine for personal growth, particularly when they experience how we, their adult mentors, are right there in it with them.

"What has been just as exciting as watching our girls mature as individuals and leaders is the response of the women mentors. They tell us that, while they originally believed committing to mentor these young girls for six years would be something of a chore, a long-term community obligation, they find they grow as much if not more than the girls they are mentoring. They say that what becomes most transformative is the opportunity to not only lead, but participate. As the years go by, girls who were 'students' evolve into the life-teachers."

Don't Wait Until You Retire

Forbes columnist and retirement activist Robert Laura warns: "Too often people think there is a magical world they will enter once they officially retire, which will help them do things they didn't do before they retired . . . walking every day, eating healthy, writing memoirs that turn into *New York Times* bestsellers, and so on. But there is nothing magical about retirement. In fact, it's my belief that retirement will only magnify what you already are. If you frequent the couch, prefer fatty foods, or indulge in an evening cocktail before bed, retirement will only provide more time for you to reinforce your existing habits."

CHAPTER 14

PARTNER WITH CARE

M Y PERSONAL OPINION IS THAT girlfriends and pets are
nonnegotiable companions, but most women also long for a
Prince Charming with whom to float into forever. Is marriage worth
the effort?

WHEN IT WORKS

Phyllis Tousey was explaining to me why she is convinced women
should regard "breakfast and sleep as a holy disciplines," when her
phone buzzed.

"Oh my goodness," she girly-gushed, "it's Chip."

Chip is Phyllis's husband of forty-something years. He is also a
top-notch estate lawyer. I should know. He is ours.

Nothing about Phyllis makes you think "girly-gush." As a nurse
epidemiologist, her research in how nutrition and lifestyle choices
impact the immune system is rubber-hits-the-road stuff. As a

woman, her faith frames her as a no-nonsense, rock-solid pillar of her church community. So perhaps you can imagine my surprise when I watched her scramble to answer her phone, then blush as she and Chip set the time and place for their dinner date. She hung up, looked at me, and said, "He is such a blessing."

Dr. Cathy Christie shared, "I am married to the love of my life. When we are separate during our days, I can't wait until the time we are together again."

Donna Orender took the theme of happily ever after to a whole new level: "MG is my beloved."

These women, all role models for an aging experience any woman would aspire to, include a happy marriage as part of their health and beauty regimen. Medical science says they are on the right track.

HEALTH BENEFITS OF MARRIAGE

Research suggests that married people enjoy significantly better health than the unmarried. In other words, marriage is good for your health and your heart, in more ways than one. In fact, one sociologist suggested the health benefits of marriage are as significant as the benefit from giving up smoking. Here are top findings:

Married adults have a greater likelihood of living longer than their unmarried counterparts. Married people live longer because they are more likely to enjoy better physical health. This is partly due to the fact they're more likely to recognize symptoms, seek medical treatment, avoid risky behavior, recover quicker, and eat a healthier diet. Spouses are intimately aware of and impacted by their spouse's choices. In a sense, couples have a significant vested interest in watching out for one another and encouraging healthy choices and behavior. Researchers found emotional support from a spouse can help people recover from both minor and major illnesses and even help cope with chronic diseases. Some studies even suggest that marital relationships actually boost the immune system, making sickness less likely in the first place.

Married women are less likely to suffer from any form of mental illness. Married people have significantly lower rates of severe depression and at least half the likelihood of developing any psychiatric disorder than never-married, cohabiting, and divorced people. According to Tara Parker-Pope, the Well columnist for the *New York Times* and author of *For Better: The Science of a Good Marriage*, some of today's most interesting research on the relationship between marriage and health is being led by a pair of researchers at Ohio State University College of Medicine. The duo, Ronald Glaser and Jan Kiecolt-Glaser, are also, fittingly, married to each other. Glaser and Kiecolt-Glaser's scholarly collaboration has its roots in a chance encounter during a faculty picnic in October 1978 on the Ohio State campus. Glaser and Kiecolt eventually met for lunch at the university's hospital cafeteria. They married a year later, in January 1980.

Recruiting seventy-six women—half of whom were married and the other half separated or divorced—the Glasers used marital-quality scales, types of questionnaires that ask couples to indicate agreement or disagreement with statements like "If I had to do it over again, I would marry the same person" or "We often do things together."

Next, using blood tests, the Glasers measured the women's immune-system responses, tracking their levels of antibody production and other indicators of immunity strength. The results showed that the women in unhappy relationships and the women who remained emotionally hung up on their ex-husbands had decidedly weaker immune responses than the women who were in happier relationships (or were happily out of them).

AN UNHAPPY MARRIAGE CAN MAKE YOU SICK

Research shows that women in an unhappy marriage have a weaker immune system than women who are happily married or divorced. Marriage stress and heart problems have a strong connection with women. Women who face the highest level of stress in marriage increase the possibility of a heart attack and bypass.

Relationship stress can also affect the body's ability to heal. In the research, wounds took a day longer to heal with partners who quarreled compared to those who didn't. With couples who showed a higher tension and a high level of hostile behavior, the wounds took two days longer to heal.

HAPPILY EVER AFTER HITS A SNAG
FOR THE OVER-FIFTY CROWD

Married women should face the fact that odds are that they will someday be alone. Across the industrialized world, women still live five to ten years longer than men. Among people older than 100 years old, 85 percent are women. And while widowhood might loom, new research from the National Center for Family and Marriage Research at Bowling Green University in Ohio shows that one in four people getting divorced is older than fifty. In 1990, the statistic was less than one in ten.

According to the Modeling Income in the Near Term (MINT)

data system, divorced and widowed baby boomer women are one of the fastest growing economically vulnerable population segments. Women who choose to think their husbands, or any man, will take care of them financially for life are engaged in highly risky thinking.

The scenarios for risk and naïveté vary. There are women who continue to rely on a spouse as their sole financial safety net, other women who consider how best to merge investment portfolios should they marry again, and a burgeoning subset of breadwinning women who need to protect personal assets in the event of divorce. Yes, breadwinning women.

A 2012 survey of 1,410 American women and 604 men—between the ages of twenty-five and sixty-eight—found that 53 percent of women make more money than their male counterparts, with an increasing number of women assuming this role as a result of partners losing jobs during the financial crisis, divorce, and marrying later in life.

KEEP DOLLARS IN YOUR OWN POCKET

In 2006, Kristen Walter was living her dream life. Her college-sweetheart-turned-husband Scott adored her. Their two children, Nick and Lexi, were healthy, good kids. Scott's executive level job allowed a nice house in friendly community with country club amenities. Kristen loved being the mom who kept their home sparkling with good energy and home-cooked meals while also serving as room mom, softball coach, and Bible study leader.

Then disaster struck. Scott, only thirty-seven at the time, woke up having a massive heart attack. Blessfully, Scott recovered but a few months later he rocked Kristen's world again saying:

"Honey, we need to think about you doing something."

Kristen says, "I remember that moment vividly. I was standing at our kitchen sink washing dishes. My gut hurt. The idea of working outside our home was as foreign to me as standing on a street corner hustling. But, though I wanted to ignore him, I knew in my heart Scott was right. I prayed and asked for guidance. Because family was and is my priority, I asked God to help me plan my life around my work, not my work around my life."

Soon after, Kristen met Molly Geil, executive national vice president for Arbonne International, in the grocery line. One friendly conversation spawned more. Soon Kristen was in the business of marketing beauty, health, and wellness products to women. In eight months, she had earned an Arbonne Mercedes-Benz. Amazingly, her team was able to do this in Nevada, which at the time was the hardest-hit state in the recession.

Avoid the Gilded Cage

Fifteen minutes late, Lauren swept into the Palm wearing a vintage cream-colored Chanel confetti skirt suit and gold Fendi kitten heels. Heads turned. Zigzagging through white tablecloths, handing out business cards right and left, Lauren was her own best advertisement.

Spotting Sandy, Lauren shimmied into a corner booth. "How are you, sweetie?" she asked, leaning in for a kiss while surreptitiously scrutinizing her oldest friend.

"Fine, good," Sandy answered, then nervously looked at her watch.

Antennae up, Lauren schmoozed on. "And how's Dan? Any news from his last interview?"

"Dan? Well . . . Dan's fine. Just a little depressed. But that's normal, you know. He's been chief operating officer of a multimillion dollar company for years. How do you stop that one day and start inter-viewing the next?"

Their waiter interrupted. Lauren ordered a bottle of Groth Char-donnay. Sandy demurred at first but, when the wine was poured, gulped almost the entire glass in one swallow.

"Honey," Lauren cooed, "you look a little thin. Eat some bread."

"Oh, I've been running more. With Dan in the house all the time, he keeps the television blaring and it makes me nervous. So I go running two to three times a day now. Dan doesn't mind. He likes me thinner."

Despite layers of silver and diamond bangles, Lauren noticed a purplish smudge around Sandy's right wrist. "Is Dan drinking more?" she probed gently.

Sandy's nose flared like a spooked thoroughbred. "Not really. I mean, he never has a scotch before five. An occasional Bloody Mary in the morning and maybe some wine with lunch, but that doesn't count when you are essentially on eternal vacation. I mean, look at us." She tipped her wineglass in Lauren's direction.

Lauren had gleaned enough. Seven years earlier, she had walked out with her three teenage girls, cash in wallet, and as much clothes and jewelry as could be stuffed into the back of her BMW sedan. Des-perate for funds, she staged a couture consignment sale at a friend's house four states away. To her amazement, she scored four thousand dollars, which she immediately reinvested shopping at estate sales and, later, rifling through European flea markets.

Today she owns Couture Closets in five cities, a wonderful river-front home in town, and a dream-retreat cabin outside of Asheville. Best of all, all three daughters were in college on her dime, not a penny required from their scumbag father.

"Sandy," she said now, "I could truly use your help. Please become one of my buyers. You would be great. We would have such fun traveling to estate sales all over the world. It would be like old times when we stewed for Delta. Best of all, think how great it would be making your own money finding fabulous clothes!"

SOMETIMES PRINCE CHARMING FARTS

"Genie, are ya'll hiring at the medical practice? I have a friend who really needs a job."

Ughhh. I hate being buttonholed by friends with unskilled children, relatives, or chums needing work. Nevertheless, every so often a pearl lands in my lap.

"We are recruiting for a position in our front office, Sue. Tell me about your friend."

"She is absolutely amazing. She has chaired four events for the school where my Brian is and each one blew the roof off fundraising. I don't know how she does it with three children in three different schools, but she is equally active with all of them and also last year chaired the board of Girls, Inc. I know from experience that she is fanatically organized, always working off lists and spreadsheets. And she is an excellent writer. You wouldn't believe the quarterly fund-raising updates she sends out mixing facts and figures with true-to-life stories. But she's no nerd. She has a super laugh and a really sweet way of encouraging others to do their best. When Marilynne chairs an event, the other moms can't move fast enough to sign up for her committees."

Hmmm. Goal-oriented lists and spreadsheets, chairing a nonprofit board, strong writing skills, proven motivational talent, a good sense of humor and—evidently—superior time management abilities . . . I was intrigued.

"What's her name again?"

"Marilynne Ford. Her husband was Chris Ford."

"Chris Ford the Ponte Vedra stockbroker who supposedly put on an Armani suit, drank a bottle of Dom Perignon, and drove his Porsche off the Dames Point Bridge?"

"Uh-huh."

Three days later I interviewed Marilynne. She was candid that, while she had not worked for pay in close to twenty years, her family's recent tragedy meant she now had to. She was poised and articulate. Most impressive was her clear determination to provide her children with an alternate example of how to cope when times are tough.

I didn't hire her. Instead, I passed her résumé onto the chair of a search committee. Within six weeks, Marilynne was named development coordinator for Experience Works, a nonprofit organization committed to helping older adults re-enter the workforce.

WHEN THE GOING GETS TOUGH, REMEMBER WHY YOU FELL IN LOVE

When Smiles first introduced me to Randy on Christmas Eve 2002, I hardly noticed him. He was nice enough, and I loved his two-year-old lab, Rigger, but I was relishing my time alone and not interested in men or dating.

After that, Randy came back and forth from Jacksonville to Apalachicola almost every weekend. I would see him when the three of us—Smiles, Randy, and I—would have dinner. I slowly became intrigued by this gentle, gifted healer who paradoxically was also a good old boy who loved to hunt and fish.

On May 7, 2003, we went to lunch. Alone. As Smiles used to say, "Randy came home from that lunch thirty-six hours later."

Not long after, I moved to Jacksonville. Three years later, we married.

What's funny about Randy and me is that our paths have always been very close. I grew up in Panama City, Florida, only an hour and a half away from Apalachicola. We shopped at the same store for our Easter outfits, our parents celebrated special occasions at the same small Italian restaurant, and we believe we vacationed on St. George Island only blocks away from each other at least three times.

What's real about the two of us is that we share a deep faith in God. We also both understand the importance of family, blood and chosen. We are quirky, jointly spoiling our blended pet family— Rigger, Bodhi, and Nami—as if they are baby angels. And, not to be understated, we have both been healthcare mavericks, ahead of our time in our individual and shared commitment to a more integrated, holistic model of care. But these last several years we have hit some rough waters.

"Rough as in the size of a puddle?" my friend Deirdre asked.

"More like the size of the Atlantic Ocean. But we hung in there."

"What helped you weather the storm?"

"After another same-theme fight, I was majorly upset, stressed, and sleepless. About three in the morning I got up and started working on my computer. Work is my go-to drug to dull anything I don't want to feel or can't figure out. Randy came downstairs, and instead of ridiculing me for being an over-the-top workaholic or starting up our fight again, he popped a bottle of champagne, poured me a glass, turned on that Cajun redneck reality show *Duck Dynasty*, and suggested I curl up with him to watch. I was so surprised I did.

"Something happened that night. As we laughed, sipped, and cuddled, I remembered why I fell in love with this man—not as a doctor or my business partner but as a guy. Just a goofy, sometimes selfish, yet pretty sexy guy who happens to really love me.

"The next day I determined to shift my attention away from what Randy wasn't doing for me and focus more on what I needed to do for myself. I decided to practice what I was preaching in my writing. I got back into the routine of working out regularly and scheduling time with my girlfriends. I also decided to stop bitching at Randy and hire a handyman and an executive assistant."

CHAPTER 15

MATTER, NO MATTER YOUR AGE

*There is a special place in hell for women
who do not help other women.*

—Madeleine K. Albright

EIGHTY-ONE-YEAR-OLD CAROL BARAS lives in San Diego. Over a forty-year career, Carol and her husband Bill started and ran multiple companies; some expanded into global markets. She also founded a nonprofit telephone hotline for troubled youth for which she was featured in *People* magazine and on *Good Morning America*. Over a chocolate martini, Carol told me she has "so much more left to give" and is "looking forward to what the next ten years might surprise me with."

Like Carol, you and I can choose to believe that we can make a difference. Choosing to matter means we stay needed, interesting, and relevant. No matter our age, life can matter more.

VOLUNTEER

In December 2011, I sat down with Crissy Haslam, the First Lady of Tennessee. I went to Emory University with Crissy and Bill (Governor Haslam); in fact, Crissy was a Kappa Alpha Theta sorority sister, and I was also a little sister in Bill's Sigma Chi fraternity, but it had been decades since we connected. Prettier than Sissy Spacek, with girl-next-door charm belying an astute, nimble brain, Crissy was born to be a First Lady. I asked my old friend how she hoped to use their conjoined political platform to make a difference for women and girls in Tennessee.

Crissy talked about Bill's linked commitment to improving education and adding jobs across the state. She described her own passion for early literacy improvement, the importance of coaching parents as to the exponential benefits of reading with their children, and how she hoped to help catalyze more parental involvement in schools. Crissy was articulate and eloquent. Then I asked, "How do you make it real? Your philanthropic interests, I mean?"

Crissy's eyes lit up. She leaned forward, becoming immediately animated, talking with her hands and punctuating certain sentences with a tap of her foot. She told me about delivering meals for the Love Kitchen, a nonprofit in Knoxville, Tennessee, that provides meals, clothing, and emergency food packages to the homebound, homeless, and unemployed. She beamed, explaining how the Love Kitchen was founded by two retired grandmothers and sisters, Helen

Ashe and Ellen Turner, who felt God placed in their hearts a mission to serve via food for the hungry.

"For decades I served on multiple nonprofit boards, and, of course, Bill and I regularly tithed to church and many charitable organizations," Crissy shared, "but it wasn't until I personally picked up those meals, drove, delivered them, and looked into the eyes of those I was serving that I truly felt it—you know, the reality of what my time commitment on boards really meant, and also the pay-it-forward value of the checks we write. My experience made me humble. It made my privilege to give intensely, intimately real."

GIVE WISELY

Women have for centuries been the fuel of our nation's volunteer efforts; now we are also the rising force in philanthropy. According to Betsy Brill, founder of Strategic Philanthropy Ltd., and a regular contributor to Forbes.com, "It's not just *who* gives that is changing—there is, after all, a rich history of high-profile women contributing generously to significant causes—it's *how* women and *to whom* women are giving that is redefining contemporary philanthropy.

"To a great degree, the charitable giving by women, directly or through women's funds, focuses on improving the quality of life and opportunity for girls and women. The exponential growth of women's funds suggests an increasing acceptance of the idea that philanthropic investments in women and girls will increasingly fuel positive change in communities. It also suggests a growing interest in philanthropic models that allow donors to leverage and pool their charitable dollars to achieve maximum impact."

In compassionate hands, tools of influence and power can be life-giving and world-changing. Since our grandmothers marched as suffragettes and our mothers dipped their toes in the women's movement by choosing to work and demanding separate checking accounts, women across the globe have emerged as an economic force to be reckoned with. In 2009, women controlled an estimated 27 percent, about $20 trillion, of the world's wealth. Women now own more than 17 million US businesses and control $4.3 trillion of the $5.9 trillion in US consumer spending. Projections are that women-controlled wealth in the United States will grow at an average of 8 percent through 2014—making US women the largest single economic force in the world.

Absurdly, women living in the United States today are poorer than men in all racial and ethnic groups. In 2008, more than half the 37 million Americans living in poverty were women. More recent surveys tell us that 38 percent of women thirty to fifty-five years old are worried they will live at or near poverty because they cannot adequately save for retirement. Thirteen percent of women older than seventy-five are poor, compared to 6 percent of men. More bad news: poverty rates for males and females living in the United States are the same throughout childhood but increase for women during their childbearing years and again in old age.

Frankly, these facts about intractable female poverty across the globe should startle those of us who are more fortunate to action. We will be—we must be—the force narrowing this wealth-to-poverty gap.

In the United States, key findings of a 2009 report released by the Foundation Center and the Women's Funding Network included:

- Private and community foundations increased their giving for activities targeting women and girls from an estimated $412.1 million in 1990 to nearly $2.1 billion in 2006.
- Women's funds are guided by the principle that women catalyze and lead the way to change in neighborhoods and communities; 98 percent of the women's funds surveyed indicated that achieving social change was a high priority for their fund.
- Excitedly, women-led philanthropy is seeding sustainable change for women and girls, not only in this nation but across the globe. At the September 2011 Asia-Pacific Economic Cooperation summit, Secretary of State Hillary Clinton declared a tipping point for women. She said, "When we liberate the economic potential of women, we elevate the economic performance of communities, nations, and the world. There is a stimulative ripple effect that kicks in when women have greater access to jobs and the economic lives of our countries: Greater political stability. Fewer military conflicts. More food. More educational opportunity for children. By harnessing the economic potential of all women, we boost opportunity for all people."

Organizations such as the International Network of Women's Funds, the Global Fund for Women, and Women for Women International are driving a more comprehensive approach to social change by focusing philanthropic giving on initiatives impacting human rights, health, and economic empowerment—one girl or woman at a time.

Choosing where and to whom to give your hard-earned (or inherited) money, as well as where you choose to invest your precious time and individual talents, is a really big deal. I choose based on the following four criteria:

1. A cause for women, girls, or animals about which I am personally passionate,
2. Confidence/trust in the administration and leadership of that cause,
3. The pressing needs in my community that I can somehow personally impact/influence and, most important,
4. What need touches my heart as exceptionally "real."

I believe women's fingerprints on the changes we impact must be sealed with a commitment far beyond charity. Our giving is more than an academic, do-good, slam-dunk exercise. Our philanthropy must be a conscious, intellectually vetted, yet heart-driven investment.

I urge you to find a cause you are passionate about, then touch and feel that need. Like the Velveteen Rabbit, then and only then will your giving become real. Then and only then will we, as women, become the turbochargers for the change our world needs now.

LOG ON WITH PURPOSE

No matter her age, a woman wearing jeans, sitting on her patio, and typing on her iPad has the potential to have as much—if not more—impact as a herd of Capitol Hill lobbyists or a billion-dollar multimedia advertising campaign. Let men play video games. Women will tune in, log on, and make a difference. Internet and social media platforms put exponential power at our fingertips. Applications such as Facebook, Twitter, Pinterest, and blogs increasingly catapult every-day people into dynamo activists. *The Dragonfly Effect,* by Jennifer Aaker and Andy Smith, is a stimulating and inspirational resource for any woman wanting to log on, join the conversation, and have impact locally, nationally and/or globally.

One of my favorite examples of one person tapping the power of the Internet to circumvent the status quo is Chase Adams, cofounder of Watsi (watsi.org). Chase was a Peace Corps volunteer in Costa Rica when a woman on a bus approached him and asked for money to help fund her son's needed medical treatment. Chase told me he "had an epiphany" and soon returned to the States with the mission of developing a crowd-funding community to connect people like you and me with patients in serious need of medical care and treatments.

In summer 2012, only two years after Chase's original epiphany, his vision went live, relying fully on volunteer talent. Neera was one of the first patients funded on Watsi. She is a twenty-four-year-old Nepali woman who had suffered from seizures since she was a child. Her mother died when she was young and her father remarried, but Neera was never taken to seek treatment for her condition. Neera was later married and then widowed, a position that carries major social stigma in Nepal. One day, while Neera was cooking (a task that Nepali women are expected to perform regardless of ability) she had a seizure and suffered severe burns on her face and body.

When Neera's profile was posted on Watsi, she needed skin graft-ing and reconstructive surgery to repair severe damage caused by burns. Neera comes from a district in Nepal where the average per capita income is less than a dollar a day. She had no financial support from her family and could not afford the $975 medical treatment she needed. She was literally out of options.

Then, something amazing happened. Twenty-two Watsi donors stepped in and fully funded Neera's treatment. Now, for the first time in four years, Neera has regained the use of her hand. Her burns have been treated and her skin is healing. She is on track to live a normal, happy, healthy life.

Cecelia is a Watsi donor. When asked, "Why do you support Watsi and why did you share it on Facebook?" here's what she said: "I'm a two-time breast cancer survivor. I have the wonderful First World benefit of insurance, a good job led by supportive people, a husband who makes enough to give me the room to take care of myself . . . in short, I'm rich beyond measure compared to almost everyone else in the world. I have so much to be grateful for."

"Every day I get piles and piles and piles of mail from nonprofits looking for money. I don't blame them—I know times are tough. I've worked for nonprofits before and I know how things work. But it hasn't stopped my becoming inured to the pleas. It's like walking down a street with hundreds of hands in my way, and I've started to feel resentful. Because of my experience, I know that the mailers I'm getting cost money, and that some of these organizations are only passing a small percentage of the donations they receive to the actual people they're purporting to help."

"Along comes Watsi, allowing me to donate directly to someone in need. And there she is—a sixty-year-old woman facing cancer and the debilitating treatments on her own, without all my resources. And all my money goes to her treatment. Alleluia! Thank you for allowing me to share."

Unfortunately, the misconception persists that technology-based communication is primarily a playground for the young-in-years. This is dead-wrong thinking. A growing composite of data from such respected sources as the American Association of Retired Persons (AARP) and the Pew Research Foundation indicates that the over-fifty crowd is one of the fastest growing segments using mobile technology. And, according to Facebook, since 2008 the number of women over fifty-five on the site has tripled and makes up the social network's fastest-growing age-group.

Slow to enter the world of social media, I attended the 2012 BlogHer conference in New York. I hated to miss the wave of our future but, like many other women, my concern was time. With everything else on my to-do list, when was I supposed to tweet or whatever? Deanna Zandt, author of *Share This!* shot back: "Social networking is much more than a way to find your high school friend or learn what your favorite celebrity had for breakfast. It's how women can connect, share our stories, and build empathetic relationships that change our world. But the world needs many different kinds of voices to make these conversations work. We need you!"

Soon after, while speaking to a group of seventy-something women, I asked them how many had an opinion regarding pro-choice movements.

"Do you mean how many of us are for it?" one woman asked crisply.

"No, how many of you have an opinion one way or another?"

All forty-two hands shot up.

"You may have read recently that thousands of Turkish women rallied in Istanbul amid growing fears that the Turkish Islamic government might ban abortion. Whether you are pro-choice or pro-life, you can have a voice in this controversy. All you have to do is log on."

Three days later, seventy-nine-year-old Anne sent me this e-mail: "After hearing you speak, I logged on and joined in several blog conversations. I also asked my thirty-four-year-old granddaughter to help me set up a Twitter account and teach me how to tweet. She got my thirteen-year-old-great-granddaughter involved. For the first time in decades, they looked at me as if I was interesting, as if I had something to say. Now my fifty-six-year-old daughter is envious of their attention and praise. She asked me if I would show her how to log on and join in too. Thank you for reminding me that my voice matters, that someone out there still cares to hear what I have to say."

Vote and/or Run

Twenty-three-year-old Lacey walked from the den where her father Lester was pumping his fists in the air watching Fox News talking heads on his wide-screen TV into the sunroom where her mother, Ronnie, sat highlighting "The National Women's Political Caucus Guide for How to Run Low-Budget Campaigns." Exasperated, she interrupted.

"Doesn't it seem like both of you are wasting tons of energy? I mean, both of you are passionate about opposing political agendas. Why get so worked up? At the end of the day, you will just cancel out each other's vote. Why even bother?"

Ronnie faced her daughter square on.

"Why vote?" She spoke quietly but with fire, "Because my opinion matters to the future of the United States of America as well as our country's global agenda. So does your dad's. So does yours. A person's vote is not right or wrong. It is simply their voice, their personal power of truth to share and, in the process of voting, conglomerate with all the other voices in our nation. A vote is how each of us can exercise our freedom and also fulfill our responsibilities as a citizen. One person's voice can and never will cancel out another's."

"Lacey, honey, political agendas and their associated candidates will come and go. Sometimes we elect clowns, charlatans, and suited-up bags of gas, but in this nation and in our world, new voices are emerging—voices of activism, entrepreneurship, and compassionate capitalism. Voices with the power to change our world. Increasingly, these are the voices of women coming from the grass roots."

"Your dad's and my disparate political views have strengthened, rather than frayed, our mutual esteem of each other's intelligence and experience. Again, if you think our individual votes cancel each other out, you are dead wrong. Standing firm in our own truths while respectfully agreeing to disagree is the stuff of democracy. I suggest you reframe your experience of our family political landscape and realize that the essence of world peace is modeled in your very own home!"

Yes, your vote matters, so never, ever fail to fill out that ballot. But some of us may choose to do more. The number of women stepping up and running for office is increasing. Wonderful news: more and more of us are winning. In 2011, US women held 90, or 16.8 percent, of the 535 seats in the 112th US Congress; 17, or 17.0 percent, of the 100 seats in the Senate; and 73, or 16.8 percent, of the 435 seats in the House of Representatives. In addition, three women served as delegates to the House from Guam, the Virgin Islands, and Washington, DC. Around the world, 19.2 percent of all national parliamentary positions (including seats in the upper house or Senate, where applicable) are held by women. Of the 181 countries for which data was provided, the United States ranked almost exactly in the middle: 92nd, just above Turkmenistan.

Worried that there are not enough hours in the day for you to take care of your own health, attend to your family, grow your business or expand your career, manage your financial well-being, and also run for office? Listen to someone who is doing it to tell you that, if this is the role the Universe is calling you to fill in our world today, you can:

Last year, I gave birth to my son Joaquín—who is now nine months old. It put me in an exclusive group; I became only the eighth member of Congress to give birth while serving in office. The first woman to give birth while in office was Yvonne Braithwaite Burke in 1973. From 1973 to 1996, there were no women in Congress who gave birth! It's obvious that having a child while being responsible to thousands of constituents is a daunting task. But it's not impossible.

Not only was I able to continue serving the interests of my constituents during my pregnancy, I even made it down to the House floor—maternity gear and all—to cast votes the night before I gave birth. I'm not going to tell you it was easy. I have a great staff and a wonderful family who made it easier. If anything, this opportunity showed me how much women can accomplish.

Last fall, Stanford and the University of Chicago conducted a study comparing female lawmakers to their male counterparts. The study focused on three specific measurements of the effectiveness of each member of Congress: (1) the number of pieces of legislation each member introduced, (2) the number of members of Congress who cosponsored each piece of legislation, and (3) the amount of discretionary spending each member was able to direct to his or her district.

The conclusion of the study was clear: women are more effective legislators than men. Quantitatively, women introduce more legislation and procure more resources for their districts. Qualitatively, the legislation women introduce receives greater support from their colleagues.

The results reaffirm a truth I've seen again and again in my life and my time in Congress: women get things done and don't take no for an answer. That's not to diminish the impact of my male colleagues, but there are times when women show greater fortitude and a stronger commitment than our male counterparts. We've had to work harder to get where we are, which means we keep digging and trying new methods until we get the results we want.

Women often view issues with a 360-degrees lens—by examining parts of the debate the way it relates to the whole. Moms, aunts, sisters, or mothers in Congress are good for our government and good for our nation. It leads to better policies, better laws, and better governance. It's why our nation's Capitol now has more bathrooms for women and a breast-feeding room.

In your own day-to-day lives, you will bring out your passion for people and the world around you. Don't just sit on the sidelines. Don't just take the world as you find it. Use your voice to stand up to injustice. Empower the powerless.

You can write the laws rather than react to them. You can ensure the next generation of women legislators have an easier road and more role models than your generation does—and than my generation had.

I look forward to hearing more voices of women in the debates that will help shape the world in which my son grows up.

Excerpted from Congresswoman Linda T. Sánchez's, February 25, 2010, blog. Congresswoman Sánchez represents the 39th Congressional District of California.

THIS ONE'S FOR THE GIRLS

I don't have children of my own. I would have particularly loved to have had a daughter but not especially one with any of the men I hung out with during my procreating years. While this fact saddens me it also deepens my commitment to positively contribute to girls' lives, those belonging to women in my circle of friends, my community, and our country. How else will I live on? What better legacy could I leave?

Whenever I have a "George Bailey moment" (the character in the movie *It's a Wonderful Life* who doesn't think his life matters and considers suicide only to be interrupted by a guardian angel), I stop and consider:

I have a few fingerprints on Sarah White's life, and she many on mine. At eighteen, Sarah is already proving herself to be a committed engine for equality and social justice.

My niece Shelley recently sent me a card inscribed with the following Marianne Williamson quote:

Our deepest fear is not that we are inadequate. Our deepest fear is that we are powerful beyond measure. We ask ourselves, who am I to be brilliant, gorgeous, talented, fabulous? Actually, who are you not to be? We were born to make manifest the glory of God that is within us. And as we let our own light shine, we give other people permission to do the same.

"Genie," Shelley wrote inside, "you teach me this. I would not be who I am or be excited about the woman I will continue to grow into without you in my life." Hardly a better legacy than that, except possibly . . .

I adore Randy's daughter Danika and am goo-goo for our granddaughter Lulu. I am sure I will spoil her, but more than that, I want to do everything I can to help her grow into a woman who is smart, strong, kind, and bold.

Besides being a super aspiration for Lulu, "Smart, strong, and bold" is the motto for Girls Inc. This nonprofit organization works in communities across the United States to inspire girls to be strong, smart, and bold through life-changing programs and experiences that help girls navigate gender, economic, and social barriers. I am on the board of the Girls Inc. chapter in Jacksonville, Florida. It, and the Girls Inc. chapters in Nashville, Tennessee, and Northwest Oregon are three of my personal choice philanthropies.

EPILOGUE

"**I** NEED MATCHING BRAS AND PANTIES. Really. Stop rolling your eyes and send someone. Come on. Matching bras and panties are every woman's secret empowerment."

Pause.

"Don't tell me yours don't match now?"

Trite as it sounds, I didn't know whether to laugh or cry. It was January 5, 2012. Laura had been admitted to the ICU the night before. We—Randy and I—rushed over as soon as we heard. She was supposedly "better," now in a step-down unit.

After weeks of dinosaur-heavy business stress compounded by a raw, draining, and, ultimately, pointless fight with Randy the night before, I was exhausted. Laura's hospital bed beckoned like a lemon-crème-stuffed, raspberry-iced cupcake. My foggy brain registered that coveting someone's hospital bed—particularly someone you adored—was perverse and had probably sent some weird reverberations out into the Universe.

I asked the nurse for directions to the nearest awful coffee machine and rallied, sending someone out for underwear. Excuse me, lingerie:

pastel, ultrasoft, and, of course, *matching* bras and panties.

I thought back to a night years earlier when Laura was staying with us so I could take her back and forth to Mayo for treatment. After a day of chemo-induced, dignity-stealing nausea and poopy problems, I popped a chick flick into the DVD, hoping to do something, anything, to make her smile. The movie was *Kissing Jessica Stein*. Randy was in our living room interviewing a new doctor.

If you haven't seen it, this movie is about a straight Jewish girl who becomes smitten with an elfin free spirit, who happens to also be a girl. The unlikely protagonist navigates the horror-heartbreak-acceptance of her family, as well as an unexpected rekindled attraction to her college boyfriend. It is funny. Laura and I laughed so hard Randy poked his head in.

"Can you two please be a little less loud? I am in a very serious meeting."

We put our hands over our mouths. Laura's giggles spilled like jelly beans out of an open bag. I chortled so hard wine spewed up and out my nose. Peeking around Randy, I saw Rigger, our yellow lab, licking the doctor's left ear while Nami attacked his shoelaces as if they were squirming earthworms. I barely made it to the bathroom.

It's a family trait, not incontinence . . . Sheila and I both tinkle in our panties when we belly laugh.

Randy banged the door.

Later, part bewildered, part petulant, he said, "Sometimes you act like you love Laura more than me."

Now if any weird thought just flipped across your smutty little mind, squash it.

Truth is, I did love Laura powerfully, in deep ways I cannot explain. I suppose I should have been jealous because of her history with

Randy, and also because she was a showstopper: a mix of Julianne Moore and Diane Lane good looks with a petite, sculpted figure Barbie would have envied. But Laura was so much more.

Laura was a spiritual rule-keeper, an extravagant mother, and the kind of optimist who believed Lassie would always come home before the credits rolled. To me, she was always abundantly kind, unswervingly encouraging. Laura told me I was smart, I was loved, I was on the right path. On good days, I believed her.

When I first moved in with Randy, it was Laura who counseled me on shifting from singledom to couplehood with a sense of humor in tow. She taught me mnemonics to keep straight the names of everyone in his large Catholic family. She also grooved on my work, taking notes when I described my latest team-building initiative, clipping articles on customer service and proffering stringent feedback when she thought I was too soft—or too hard—a leader.

Always feminine and gleefully accessorized, Laura teased me to be more girly. She told me to wear a lace camisole under my pinstripe suit and try honey-warm highlights around my face. She would dare me to skinny-dip and surprise Randy when he came out to walk our dogs.

Our last afternoon together, Laura urged me to learn to speak Italian, try dark chocolate with caramel and sea salt, and—of all things—make sure our medical practice did not give up converting from paper-based medical charts to electronic health records (EHR).

"I know it's expensive, Genie," she said, "and surely it's going to be a hassle, but look . . ." Laura opened a four-inch, three-ring binder showing me pages and pages of crisp, texted health records, most highlighted, some with her lusciously penciled notes and intricate drawings in the margin.

New government regulations were requiring that all hospitals and doctors' offices shift to EHR or be subject to financial penalties. But the transition was a huge investment and, understandably, Randy preferred his tried-and-true pen and paper chart to a computer keyboard and screen. I sighed.

"And this new book you are writing on aging, how's it going?"

"I am thinking of punting the whole project. There are so many books about aging already out there. Health Communications Inc. has agreed to publish, but I'll be funding a lot of the marketing and media out of pocket.

"I sit at the computer and stare at the screen for hours. I'm beginning to think the whole idea is just another ego trip, my wanting to pretend I have answers I don't. I mean, what fresh thing do I have to say about aging? It's not like I'm the poster woman for getting it right."

Laura's prednisone-puffy face sharpened. Her near-skeletal little hands reached out and grabbed mine.

"You must write this book. You have to. For Danika. For my granddaughters yet to be born."

Tears rolled down my face and off my chin.

"Promise me," she demanded.

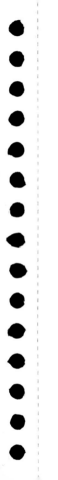

APPENDIX A:
BELLY FLAT RECIPES

Breakfast

BROILED GRAPEFRUIT   Serves 2

1 grapefruit

1 teaspoon ground ginger

1 tablespoon honey

Preheat the broiler.

Cut the grapefruit in half and use a small serrated knife to cut out the sections. Spoon the sections and juice into a bowl. Scrape out all of the remaining thick skin and pulp and discard. Spoon the sections from the bowl back into the halves. This is best done one half at a time.

Sprinkle the ginger and drizzle the honey over the top of each grapefruit half. Place the halves on a baking sheet.

Broil for 3 to 5 minutes, until the honey begins to bubble.

BANANA IN BARK   Serves 1

1 tablespoon ground almonds

1 tablespoon ground or milled flaxseed

1 whole banana

Mix almonds and flaxseeds on a large plate.

Peel banana and roll in mixture until fully covered.

Either eat immediately or place on wax paper and put in refrigerator to chill before eating.

ASPARAGUS OMELET   Serves 2

4 egg whites

¼ teaspoon salt

4 egg yolks

Dash of pepper

1 cup 1% milk-fat cottage cheese

1½ tablespoons extra-virgin olive oil

6 asparagus spears, trimmed and slightly steamed

Preheat the oven to 350° F.

Beat egg whites until frothy. Add salt and beat until stiff.

Beat yolks until thick and lemon colored; add pepper and cottage cheese and beat until well blended. Fold egg whites into yolks.

Heat olive oil in a 10-inch iron skillet; pour in omelet and cook approximately 3 minutes, until the bottom is lightly browned.

Top with asparagus spears and finish cooking in the oven for 15 minutes or until a knife inserted in the center comes out clean.

CITRUS AMBROSIA   Serves 2 to 3

1 11-ounce can mandarin oranges, drained

1 pink grapefruit (or grapefruit sections in a jar, packed in juice, not syrup), cut into ½-inch pieces

2 tangerines, cut into ½-inch pieces

1 cup fresh cherries, pitted and halved

⅛ cup silvered almonds

Toss all the ingredients together and chill for 1 hour.

EGG IN A NEST   Serves 2

2 slices whole-grain bread

Extra-virgin olive oil

2 eggs

2 tablespoons grated Parmesan cheese

Red pepper flakes to taste

Turn a small glass upside down to cut a circle out of each bread slice.

Lightly coat a skillet with olive oil, place the bread slices in the skillet, and break an egg into each hole.

Cook on medium heat, turning once until the eggs are the desired firmness.

Remove from the skillet and garnish with the Parmesan cheese and red pepper flakes.

FLAXSEED AND FRUIT SMOOTHIE   Serves 1

1 cup skim milk

1 cup frozen berries

1 banana

1 cup plain low-fat yogurt

1 tablespoon flaxseed oil

1 tablespoon ground flaxseed

Combine all ingredients except flaxseed in blender. Blend well.

Pour into large glass and stir in flaxseed.

ORANGE SMOOTHIE WITH FLAXSEEDS Serves 4

1 banana

1 6-ounce can frozen orange juice concentrate

2 cups vanilla soy milk

1 teaspoon ground ginger

2 tablespoons milled flaxseeds

Place the banana, orange juice concentrate, soy milk, and ginger in a blender. Process until the ingredients are blended and smooth.

Stir in the flaxseeds and serve.

SMILEY TOAST Serves 2

1 tablespoon sesame seed butter
(may substitute almond or peanut butter)

2 slices whole-grain or whole-wheat bread, toasted

½ banana, sliced

2 dozen raisins

Spread the sesame seed butter on the warm toast.

Use the banana slices to make eyes.

Arrange the raisins in a semicircle like a smile.

YOGURT AND FRUIT PARFAIT   Serves 1

⅓ cup ground almonds

2 tablespoons ground or milled flaxseed

1 cup plain low-fat yogurt

¾ cup berries

Raw honey (optional)

In small bowl, mix almonds with flaxseed.

In parfait glass, alternately layer yogurt, berries, and almond-flaxseed mixture.

If desired, drizzle a small amount of honey on top.

CRUSTLESS CRUCIFEROUS QUICHE   Serves 6

1 cup skim or fat-free milk

6 eggs

1 cup frozen chopped spinach, thawed, drained and squeezed dry

1 cup frozen chopped broccoli (thawed, well drained)

1 finely chopped small white onion

½ cup grated mozzarella cheese

Salt and pepper to taste

Preheat oven to 425 degrees. Beat eggs and milk together until frothy. Pour into well-oiled, medium-size iron skillet. Add in veggies and onion and top with cheese. Bake for 30 minutes until top is crusty. Add salt and pepper if needed.

MAIN DISHES:

*Perfect for
Lunch or Dinner*

TURKEY AND ASPARAGUS WRAPS   Serves 4

16 asparagus spears

⅓ cup plain low-fat yogurt

1 teaspoon lemon juice

1 teaspoon curry powder

Salt and pepper to taste

1 pound deli-style turkey breast, sliced

Wash, trim, and steam asparagus spears until tender. Set aside to cool.

Mix yogurt, lemon juice, curry powder, salt, and pepper in a small bowl.

Place 2 or 3 slices of turkey on a plate. Spread with the yogurt mixture. Put asparagus spears on one end and roll up. Secure with toothpick if necessary.

Serve immediately or refrigerate.

VEGETABLE BARLEY SOUP   Serves 8

2 quarts vegetable broth

1 cup uncooked barley

2 large carrots, chopped

2 stalks celery, chopped

1 14.5-ounce can diced tomatoes with juice

1 cup cauliflower, chopped

1 cup broccoli, chopped

1 onion, chopped

3 bay leaves

1 teaspoon garlic powder

1 teaspoon salt

½ teaspoon ground black pepper

1 teaspoon dried parsley

1 teaspoon curry powder

1 teaspoon paprika

1 teaspoon Tabasco (optional)

Pour the vegetable broth into a large pot. Add the barley, carrots, celery, tomatoes, cauliflower, broccoli, beans, onions, and bay leaves.

Season with the garlic powder, salt, pepper, parsley, curry powder, paprika, and Tabasco.

Bring to a boil, then cover and simmer over medium-low heat, stirring occasionally, for at least 1 hour.

SAVORY SPINACH
AND SALMON SALAD   Serves 4

3 tablespoons orange juice

2 tablespoons low-sodium soy sauce

2 teaspoons minced fresh ginger

1 teaspoon raw honey

1½ teaspoons extra-virgin olive oil

4 (6-ounce) salmon fillets

2 cups fresh spinach, washed

½ cup mandarin orange slices

⅓ cup chopped green onions (scallions)

2 hard-boiled eggs, sliced

¼ cup ground almonds mixed with 1 tablespoon ground or
  milled flaxseed

In a small bowl, combine the orange juice, soy sauce, ginger, and honey. Whisk, gradually adding the olive oil, until well blended.

Grill, bake, or poach the salmon fillets.

Make a bed of spinach on each of four plates. Place salmon in the center of each one.

Garnish each with mandarin orange slices, scallions, and eggs. Drizzle the orange-soy sauce dressing over the entire plate and sprinkle with almond-flaxseed mixture.

GRILLED FISH WITH CITRUS MARINADE   Serves 4

¼ cup extra-virgin olive oil

2 tablespoons grapefruit juice

3 tablespoons lime juice

Salt and pepper to taste

4 (6-ounce) fish fillets

Combine olive oil, grapefruit juice, lime juice, salt, and pepper. Pour over fish and marinate in refrigerator for 2 or more hours.

Grill and serve.

NOT YOUR ORDINARY TUNA SALAD   Serves 4

1 large (12-ounce) can white albacore tuna in water

1 red pepper, chopped fine

1 yellow pepper, chopped fine

¼ cup grated green apple

⅓ cup shredded fresh cabbage

2 tablespoons plain low-fat yogurt

½ teaspoon lemon juice

½ teaspoon rice wine vinegar

Salt and pepper to taste

Mix all ingredients together in a large bowl.

Chill for at least 1 hour before serving.

CAULIFLOWER CRAB CAKES   Serves 6

2 cups crabmeat

2 cups cooked and mashed cauliflower

⅓ cup minced celery

⅓ cup minced onion

1 tablespoon parsley

2 eggs, beaten

Extra-virgin olive oil or grapeseed oil (for sautéing)

> Combine all ingredients in a large bowl, except the olive oil.
> Form into 6 patties and chill in refrigerator for at least 1 hour.
> Brown in skillet lightly coated with olive oil.

CHICKEN AND COLD RICE SALAD   Serves 10

2 cups cooked brown rice (you may use whole-grain
   minute brown rice)

2½ cups cooked chicken, cubed

1 cup broccoli florets, steamed al dente

½ cup shredded almonds

2 tablespoons minced parsley

1 cup plain low-fat yogurt

Spinach

4 tangerines

> Toss everything together in a large bowl except the spinach and
> tangerines. Chill for at least 2 hours.
> Serve on a bed of spinach and surround with tangerine slices.

GRILLED SALMON WITH DILL AND LEMON Serves 4

2 tablespoons dill

1 teaspoon garlic powder

4 tablespoons extra-virgin olive oil

2 tablespoons white wine vinegar with tarragon

Juice of 2 lemons

4 (1-inch thick) salmon steaks, 4 ounces each

Mix dill, garlic powder, olive oil, vinegar, and lemon juice. Pour mixture over salmon steaks and marinate in the refrigerator for at least 2 hours, turning at least once.

Place salmon on hot grill and cook 3–5 minutes on each side.

TURKEY, BROCCOLI, AND CASHEW ROLL-UPS Serves 2

½ pound thinly sliced roast turkey breast

1 tablespoon honey

1 teaspoon lemon juice

½ teaspoon grated fresh ginger

½ cup finely chopped steamed broccoli

¼ cup crushed cashews

On a cutting board or on wax paper, separate the turkey slices into two piles.

In a small bowl, whisk together the honey, lemon juice, and ginger, then add the broccoli and cashews.

Spread the mixture on the turkey slices, roll up, and secure with toothpicks.

QUICK TURKEY-STUFFED CABBAGE   Serves 8

1 pound ground turkey

1 large onion, chopped

1 cup brown rice, uncooked

¼ cup fresh mint, chopped, or 1 tablespoon dried mint

1 egg, beaten

2 (14-ounce) cans chicken broth

Salt and pepper to taste

2 tablespoons extra-virgin olive oil

1 medium cabbage

2 tablespoons flaxseed

Preheat oven to 350° F.

Combine the turkey, onion, rice, mint, egg, broth, salt, and pepper and sauté in olive oil until browned.

In another pot, steam the cabbage until it is slightly soft.

After the cabbage cools, cut off the bottom, peel off the leaves, and place them in a baking dish one by one.

Spoon a helping of turkey mixture onto each leaf and then roll it up.

Sprinkle with flaxseed and bake for 15–20 minutes.

VEGETABLE-STUFFED FLANK STEAK   Serves 6

2 pounds flank steak

½ cup red wine vinegar

3 cloves garlic, finely chopped

2 teaspoons dried thyme

1 cup fresh spinach

4 large carrots, boiled and cut in ½ inch pieces

1 cup sun-dried tomatoes soaked in red wine

1 small onion, thinly sliced

3 teaspoons red pepper flakes

2 tablespoons extra-virgin olive oil

1½ cups beef broth

Arrange the steak on a cutting board so that the long side is parallel to you. Using a long knife, butterfly the steak to within ½ inch of the far edge so that it opens like a book.

Pound the steak with a mallet until about ¼ inch thick. Transfer to a baking dish, poke holes in the meat, and sprinkle with the red wine vinegar, garlic, and thyme. Cover and marinate overnight.

Preheat the oven to 375° F. Put the meat on the cutting board and top with a layer of the spinach, carrots, sun-dried tomatoes, and onions. Sprinkle evenly with the red pepper flakes.

Starting with the edge closest to you, roll the meat forward to form a tight cylinder. Using kitchen twine, tie the meat at 1-inch intervals.

Heat the olive oil in a large, deep skillet or Dutch oven and sear the meat on all sides over high heat until brown.

Pour in the beef broth, then add enough water to reach about one-third of the way up the sides of the meat.

Cover, transfer to the oven, and bake until tender, approximately 2 hours.

Remove the meat and place on a clean cutting board. Let stand 10 minutes before slicing. Spoon a tablespoon of the beef broth mixture over the meat before serving.

VEGGIE BURGERS   Serves 4

1 medium onion, chopped very fine

1 medium bell pepper, chopped very fine

Extra-virgin olive oil

2 cups cooked fresh spinach, drained and chopped fine

1 cup mashed cooked cauliflower

1 can black beans, drained

1 tablespoon garlic powder

1 egg, beaten well

2 pieces whole-grain toast, crumbled fine

Salt and pepper to taste

Sauté onion and bell pepper in olive oil until onion is translucent.

When mixture has cooled, place it in a large bowl and add all other ingredients, mixing well.

Form patties and place on cookie sheet. Chill for at least 2 hours before browning in olive oil in a skillet on top of the stove, or bake at 400°F for 30 minutes.

Salads
and
Side Dishes

CRUCIFEROUS COUSCOUS   Serves 8

1 cup minced broccoli

1 cup fresh spinach

1 cup minced cauliflower

2 tomatoes, cubed

2 tablespoons minced garlic

2 tablespoons extra-virgin olive oil

3 cups water

2 cups quick-cook couscous

2 tablespoons balsamic vinegar

Salt and pepper to taste

Preheat oven to 350° F.

Mix broccoli, spinach, cauliflower, and tomatoes with garlic and 1 tablespoon of olive oil and place on a baking sheet. Bake for 15–20 minutes, until tender.

In a pot, bring water and remaining tablespoon of olive oil to a boil, add couscous and return to a boil, then remove from heat and let stand for 5 minutes. Fluff with a fork and let cool.

Place couscous on a plate and top with roasted vegetables.

Drizzle with balsamic vinegar before serving.

BEETS AND BRUSSELS SPROUTS   Serves 6

4 medium beets

10–12 Brussels sprouts

Extra-virgin olive oil

1 small white onion, peeled and sliced thin

3 tablespoons frozen orange juice concentrate

2 teaspoons grated ginger

Salt and pepper to taste

Boil beets for 45 minutes or until tender by touch with a fork; drain when done.

Remove and discard the outer leaves of the Brussels sprouts and boil them in a separate pan for 5 minutes. Drain and cut in half.

Put olive oil in skillet, sauté onion, and add beets and Brussels sprouts. Cook until warm, about 2–3 minutes, then stir in orange juice concentrate and ginger. Salt and pepper to taste.

CREAMY COLESLAW   Serves 10

4 cups shredded cabbage

1 cup grated carrots

1½ cups plain low-fat yogurt

1½ tablespoons finely chopped celery

1 teaspoon grated onion

3 tablespoons white vinegar

1 tablespoon raw honey

¾ teaspoon salt

Dash of pepper

Mix all ingredients in a large bowl and toss well.
Refrigerate for at least 2 hours before serving.

BROCCOLI AND CAULIFLOWER IN LIME DRESSING   Serves 4

1 tablespoon low-sodium soy sauce

2 teaspoons raw honey

3 tablespoons fresh lime juice

1 cup broccoli florets

1 cup cauliflower florets

Salt and pepper to taste

Red pepper flakes (optional)

Mix soy sauce, honey, and lime juice. Set aside.

Boil broccoli and cauliflower for about 5 minutes, till they are tender yet firm. Drain and toss immediately with soysauce, lime mixture. Season with salt and pepper to taste.

Sprinkle with red pepper flakes if desired.

SPICY KALE AND BEANS   Serves 8

2 cups dried black-eyed peas

1 bunch kale (about 2 pounds)

1 large onion, diced

1 tablespoon extra-virgin olive oil

2 tablespoons white vinegar

¼ teaspoon crushed red pepper (optional)

2 hard-boiled eggs, chopped

Soak black-eyed peas overnight.

The next day place the drained peas in a large saucepan, cover with water, and bring to a boil over high heat. Boil for 3 minutes.

Remove the pan from the heat, cover tightly, and let stand for 1 hour.

Wash kale, remove large stem ends, and coarsely chop the leaves.

Sauté the onion in a large skillet. Add the kale and cook for about 5 minutes, until the leaves are wilted but still bright green. Stir in black-eyed peas, vinegar, and crushed red pepper until the entire mixture bubbles with heat.

Top with the eggs before serving.

SPINACH AND FETA BROWN RICE   Serves 6

1 cup brown rice

1 cup fresh spinach leaves

2 teaspoons minced garlic

4 tablespoons low-fat feta cheese

Salt and pepper to taste

Cook the brown rice according to directions on the package, or bring to a boil 2 parts water to 1 part rice in a medium-size pot. Cook on low for 30–45 minutes until the rice is soft.

Before serving, add the spinach and garlic, stirring until the spinach wilts.

Put on a plate and garnish with feta cheese.

BEET AND ORANGE SALAD   Serves 4

1 jar pickled beets

2 cans mandarin oranges in water, or 2 tangerines,
  peeled, sectioned, and seeded

½ cup orange juice

1 cup fresh spinach

¼ cup slivered almonds

Toss beets and mandarin orange or tangerine sections in orange juice. Chill for at least 1 hour.

Serve on bed of spinach.

Garnish with slivered almonds.

MASHED CAULIFLOWER
WITH TURKEY BACON   Serves 4

1 medium head cauliflower

Salt and pepper to taste

¼ cup skim milk

¼ cup instant low-carb mashed potatoes

1 teaspoon garlic paste or garlic powder

2 slices cooked turkey bacon, crumbled

Cut cauliflower into florets and steam with salt and pepper until very tender.

Place in blender and add all ingredients except turkey bacon. Blend until smooth.

Return to pot or stove to reheat if necessary.

Garnish with crumbled turkey bacon.

CABBAGE-APPLE SALAD   Serves 6

1 cup shredded cabbage

1 cup diced apple

1 cup chopped celery

¼ cup plain low-fat yogurt

2 tablespoons flaxseed

Mix all ingredients in a large bowl. Toss, chill, and serve.

SKILLET BROCCOLI OR
ASPARAGUS WITH SESAME SEEDS Serves 6

2 large stalks fresh broccoli or 12–14 asparagus spears
2 tablespoons extra-virgin olive oil
2 tablespoons sesame seeds
2 or 3 cloves garlic, peeled and sliced
Salt and pepper to taste

Wash broccoli and cut the florets into medium to large pieces. Peel the tough outer layer from the stems and slice the inner tender, juicy portion in half.

Or, if using asparagus, wash the spears and trim off the ends.

In a large skillet with a lid, heat the oil over high heat. Add sesame seeds and sauté, stirring until lightly toasted; be careful not to overcook, because they burn quickly. Also, keep a lid handy because the sesame seeds might start to pop.

Add the broccoli (or asparagus) and garlic, and stir for a few seconds. Add salt and pepper to taste, and stir.

Cover the skillet and remove from heat; let sit about 15 minutes. The broccoli (or asparagus) will retain its color and be tender and crisp.

APPENDIX B:
RESOURCES

BEST RESOURCE: YOURSELF

YOU WANT TO MAKE SMART, belly-flat-friendly, hormone-healthy choices but may not be sure where to start. While this section provides a listing of suggested resources, I want to take a minute to remind each reader that you are the one in charge of determining what is right for you, your body, and ultimately, your health.

I strongly encourage you to do your research, ask informed questions, reach out to other women for input and vet health and medical professionals to discern their credentials, training, experience, and reputation. Ultimately assemble a health coaching and care team you trust, but remember: Even with your team in place, you are the common variable in every health and wellness conversation you will have. Therein, you must always take the lead.

CHOOSING ORGANIC

Foods

Many people initially complain that buying organic meat and produce is too expensive and that sorting through food product labels to determine GMO versus non-GMO foods can be confusing. The good news is that, because of growing consumer demand, almost every grocery store in the nation now stocks organic foods and also has a health food aisle. Some progressive grocery store chains in larger metropolitan markets even have a nutritionist on the floor available to help you sort through questions, labels, and foods to match special dietary needs.

I applaud the grocery store industry for increasingly responding to shoppers wanting more natural options. My hat is off to two companies who continue to raise the bar:

Whole Foods Markets: Founded in 1980 as one small store in Austin, Texas, Whole Foods Markets is now the world's leading retailer of natural and organic foods, with more than 340 stores in North America and the United Kingdom. This is a mission-driven company whose popularity and growth deserves celebration. To find a Whole Foods Market near you, go to www.wholefoodsmarket.com.

Trader Joe's: I particularly like the clear labeling of all Trader Joe's private labeled products clearly promising NO artificial flavors, colors or preservatives, NO monosodium glucarate (MSG), NO genetically modified (GMO) ingredients, NO added trans fats. There are currently 375 Trader Joe's grocery stores in the United States. To find one near you, go to www.traderjoes.com/stores.

To learn more about the "why" of organic food choices, or to locate a source for organic foods near you, go to: www.organicfoods.com, www.organicconsumers.org, www.eatwell.org, and www.Nutrition Style.com. Local farmer's markets can also be a great source for organic foods, often at lower prices than you will pay in the supermarket or health food store.

Housecleaning Products

Remember it is important to decrease your exposure to environmental estrogens, or xenoestrogens. I recommend using organic, eco-friendly housecleaning products when at all possible. One excellent resource is Billee Sharp's book *Lemons and Lavender.* Also check out www.greenworkscleaners.com and www.eartheasy.com.

Safe Cosmetics

I urge you to make sure your cosmetics are safe. Many are not. An excellent website for detailed information on beauty products is www.safecosmetics.org. The Campaign for Safe Cosmetics is a coalition of public health, educational, religious, labor, women's environmental and consumer groups. The coalition's goal is to require the health and beauty industry to protect consumer health by phasing out all chemical ingredients linked to cancer, birth defects, and other health problems, and replace them with safer alternatives.

If you want to learn more and then take informed action, Ellen Murmur's book *Simple Skin Beauty: Every Woman's Guide to a Lifetime of Healthy, Gorgeous Skin* is a wonderful resource. Whole Foods Premium Body Care line of products are among the most exceptional and affordable personal care products available. They meet the strictest standards for quality sourcing, environmental impact, results and safety. Whole Foods Premium Body Care is an excellent choice for being good to your whole body.

In addition, many websites inform and offer naturally terrific products. Some favorites include:

www.kellyteegardenorganics.com
www.tataharperskincare.com
www.aubrey-organics.com
www.burtsbees.com
www.dermae.com
www.pangeaorganics.com
www.weleda.com

Note: Some of these products are more wallet-friendly than others. Do your homework, check out reviews, ask for samples and, ultimately, choose the ones that work best for your body, face and budget.

Vaginal Lubricants

Over-the-counter vaginal lubricants can be a good choice to self-treat a condition of vaginal dryness, but read the label before you buy. Some ingredients in certain products are absolute no-no's because they create a medium for bacteria and growth, thereby increasing risk of urinary tract infection. Others contain potentially harmful petrochemicals. Safe sources for vaginal lubricants include:

www.bewellstaywell.com/Sylk-Natural
www.goodcleanlove.com
www.yesyesyes.org

If a condition of vaginal dryness and/or painful intercourse persists, consult your doctor.

Vitamins and Supplements

According to a recent survey of nearly 1,000 supplements conducted by ConsumerLab.com, a product-certification company, one out of four supplements has quality problems, such as contamination or a failure to include an ingredient listed on the label.

I own the Natural Medicine Pharmacy that adjoins Randy's Ageless and Wellness Medical Center. Drawing on Randy's expertise as a physician specializing in age-management medicine, as well as his training as a compounding pharmacist specializing in pharmacognosy (plant-based medicine), I have established one criterion for the vitamins and supplements we carry that is simple yet non-negotiable: **Research-driven dietary supplements with a proven track record.** This means digging deep to **evaluate quality, truth in labeling, and company adherence to stringent manufacturing guidelines.** These guidelines include:

- Raw materials testing
- Potency testing
- Product traceability
- Purity testing
- Product freshness
- Microbiology testing

The bottom line is truth in packaging. People have the right to know what they are putting in their body and they deserve to get the amount of active ingredient they are paying for. Randy has developed a signature-formulation, private-label line of vitamins and supplements available online at www.hormonewellstore.com.

Randy has also vetted and recommends the following brands. The following three are available only through a physician's office. For more information on their products or to find a doctor in your area who carries them, go to:

- Metagenics, www.metagenics.com
- Orthomolecular, www.orthomolecularproducts.com
- Xymogen, www.xymogen.com

Life Extension is a direct-to-consumer source for vitamins and supplements that Randy and I have high confidence in. In addition to its natural product offerings, Life Extension publishes a fantastic scientifically rooted monthly magazine. For more information on Life Extension, go to www.lef.org.

HORMONE HEALTH

Over-the-Counter Progesterone Creams

Many women find that using an over-the-counter (OTC) bioidentical progesterone cream is an excellent first step toward eliminating estrogen dominance and restoring hormone balance. You can purchase bioidentical progesterone creams in most health foods stores. The good news is that it is available. The bad news is that some products are better than others. The reason for this discrepancy: There is no regulatory body that oversees the production or standardization of product manufacturing for so-called "natural" products. What this means to the average consumer is that there is great variation among the many OTC progesterone creams on the market today.

While I cannot reveal Randy's exact formula for his Natural Balance Cream, I can share here several of the critical variables that define its integrity of ingredients and proven efficacy:

- Dr. Randolph's Natural Balance Cream is a bioidentical formulation of progesterone. This means that the molecules of progesterone suspended in the cream have exactly the same molecular structure as those produced by the human body. The body recognizes, receives, and utilizes these molecules. The parent molecule for progesterone comes from a substance known as diosgenin, which is found in soy or Mexican wild yam. Many products on the market today containing soy or Mexican wild yam claim to be a "natural progesterone"; however, until the diosgenin is converted from its original molecular structure, the body will not recognize it. Consequently, soy or Mexican wild yam it the raw state will not generate the same clinical response.

- Dr. Randolph's Natural Balance Cream contains the maximum concentration of bioidentical progesterone that can be mixed in an OTC product. Some creams have a "little" progesterone in their mix but not enough to generate a consistent and positive user response.

- The progesterone in Dr. Randolph's Natural Balance Cream meets the United States Pharmacopoeia gold standards for quality and purity. In addition, the laboratory used to produce Dr. Randolph's Natural Balance Cream compounds this product under strict guidelines approved by the National Association of Compounding Pharmacists. This is not required by law so not all product manufacturers go to the trouble or expense.

- The progesterone molecule in Dr. Randolph's Natural Balance Cream is encased within a liposomal delivery system. This is critical because, as the many layers of the oily globule of liposome melt away like a snowball, the hormones are dispersed continuously through the skin for up to twelve hours. This means that the underlying issue of hormonal imbalance is eliminated, hormonal balance is restored, and my patients have continuous relief of their symptoms throughout the day. In contrast, other over-the-counter progesterone creams are not formulated for sustained release. When the progesterone is immediately absorbed through the skin, a quick spike in progesterone levels occurs causing a temporary vs. constant relief of symptoms. Therein a formulation that is time-released is much more clinically effective.

Dr. Randolph's Natural Balance Cream is available at www.hormonewellstore.com. Randy has also reviewed the following OTC progesterone creams and verified their quality and truth in advertising:

Arbonne International
PhytoProlief and Prolief Natural Balancing Creams
www.arbonne.com
Emerita
Pro-Gest progesterone cream
www.progest.com

Seeking Medical Professional Help

If you have committed to the lifestyle changes outlined in this book and tried an OTC progesterone cream for more than one month with no relief of symptoms, this is a signal that your body needs more. It is time for you to seek professional medical help to diagnose and treat a more advanced or more multifactorial underlying condition of hormone imbalance.

Caution: treating hormone imbalances is serious medicine. Do your homework before choosing a medical professional. Find out:

- Board certification(s)
- Training in hormone health, what organization, how long. Excellent organizations offering continuing medical education (CME) programs on natural hormone health are the American Academy of Anti-Aging Medicine (A4M), www.a4m.com and the Institute of Functional Medicine, www.functional medicine.org
- Protocol for routinely analyzing hormone levels via blood work or saliva testing.
- Years of experience
- Reputation among patient community, then
- Trust your instincts. Is this someone you can partner with and trust?

When looking for a physician or medical professional in your area, an excellent resource can be your local compounding pharmacist. If you need help finding a compounding pharmacy in your area, contact one of the two organizations listed here.

**The International Academy of
Compounding Pharmacists (IACP)**
P.O. Box 1365
Sugar Land, TX 77487
Phone: 281-933-8400
Fax: 281-495-0602
Website: http://www.iacprx.org

Professional Compounding Centers of America (PCCA)
9901 South Wilcrest Drive
Houston, TX 77099
Phone: 877-798-3224
Fax: 877-765-1422
Website: http://www.pccarx.com

Finally, patients come to Dr. Randolph's Ageless and Wellness Medical Center from across the nation and around the globe. If you are interested in scheduling an appointment with Randy or one of the medical professionals trained by him practicing within our clinic, call (904) 249-3743 or reach us through our website, www.agelessandwellness.com.

Testing Hormone Levels

Measuring hormone levels is essential for the proper diagnoses of perimenopause, menopause, andropause, or other disease states such as hypothyroidism and adrenal exhaustion (chronic fatigue syndrome). Hormone level testing also enables your physician to closely monitor hormone levels during treatment to ensure they all remain adequately balanced and within the optimal physiological range. Hormone levels can be analyzed through blood, saliva, or urine.

Physicians on the cutting edge of optimal aging medicine are increasingly adding specialized lab services into the clinics. At Dr. Randolph's Ageless and Wellness Medical Center we have recently partnered with Atherotech Diagnostic Lab, www.atherotech.com, and Genova Diagnostics, www.gdx.net. An emerging, and still controversial, trend is lab companies offering tests directly to the consumer. Two very credible companies offering this service are:

- MyMedLab, www.mymedlab.com
- ZRT, www.zrtlab.com

Recommended Reading

Hormone Health

If you have not already done so, I strongly recommend you read the first two books Randy and I co-authored: *From Hormone Hell to Hormone Well* and *From Belly Fat to Belly Flat.* The first will provide you a more comprehensive treatise of the history and science behind bioidentical hormone replacement. The second expounds more fully on the links between estrogen dominance, belly fat, and what you can do about it. Other excellent hormone health resource books include:

Lee, John R., MD, with Virginia Hopkins. *What Your Doctor May Not Tell You About Menopause.* New York: Warner Books, 1996.

Lee, John R., MD, with Jesse Hanley, MD, and Virginia Hopkins. *What Your Doctor May Not Tell You About Perimenopause.* New York: Warner Books, 1999.

Lee, John R., MD, with David Zava, PhD, and Virginia Hopkins. *What Your Doctor May Not Tell You About Breast Cancer.* New York: Warner Books, 2002.

Morgentaler, Abraham, MD, *Testosterone for Life: Recharge Your Vitality, Sex Drive and Overall Health.* New York: McGraw Hill, 2009.

Northrup, Christiane, MD, *Women's Bodies, Women's Wisdom: Creating Physical and Emotional Health and Healing.* New York: Bantam Books, 1994.

Northrup, Christiane, MD, *The Wisdom of Menopause: Creating Physical and Emotional Health and Healing During the Change.* New York: Bantam Books, 2001.

Schwartz, Erika, MD, *The Hormone Solution.* New York: Warner Books, 2002.

Seaman, Barbara. *The Greatest Experiment Ever Performed on Women: Exploding the Estrogen Myth.* New York: Hyperion Books, 2003.

Somers, Suzanne, *Ageless: The Naked Truth About Bioidentical Hormones.* New York: Crown Publishers, 2006.

Somers, Suzanne, *The Sexy Years, Discover the Hormone Connection: The Secret to Fabulous Sex, Great Health, and Vitality for Women and Men.* New York: Crown Publishers, 2004.

Taylor, Eldred, MD, and Bell-Taylor, Ava, MD, *Are Your Hormones Making You Sick?* Physicians Natural Medicine, Inc., 2000.

Wilson, James L., ND, DC, PhD, *Adrenal Fatigue.* Petaluma, CA: Smart Publications, 2003.

REFERENCES

PROLOGUE

Crary, D. (2011, August 11). Boomers will be spending billions to counter aging. *Boston*. Retrieved from http://articles.boston.com/2011-08-20/lifestyle/29909735 _1_anti-aging-retirement-age-dietary-supplements.

INTRODUCTION

Randolph, C. W., & James, G. (2009). Chapter 1: Decades of Desperate Women Dangerously Duped. In *From Hormone Hell to Hormone Well.* (pp. 5–22). Deerfield Beach, Florida: Health Communications, Inc.

CHAPTER 1

Randolph, C. W. (2009). *From Hormone Hell to Hormone Well.* (2nd ed.). (pp. 1–240). Deerfield Beach, Florida: Health Communications, Inc.

Baron, P. (2005, June). "Hormone Testing for Optimal Health." *Life Extension Magazine*.

Hormone treatment options (2012). *Women in Balance*. Retrieved July 23, 2012, from http://womeninbalance.org/choices-in-therapy/hormone-treatment-options/.

Randolph, C. W. (2011). Women's Hormone Health. *Dr. Randolph's Natural Hormone Institute*. Retrieved July 23, 2012, from http://www.hormonewell.com/manage_moods.html.

Mayeaux, E. J. (2005, August 30). The menopausal patient and hormone replacement therapy. *LSU.* Retrieved August 25, 2012, from http://www.sh.lsuhsc.edu/fammed/outpatientmanual/menopause-hrt.htm.

"Hormone Balance." (2012, March 29). *Life Extension.*

CHAPTER 2

Weight loss in middle age. (2012). *Livestrong.* Retrieved August 3, 2012, from http://www.livestrong.com/weight-loss-in-middle-age/.

Gann, C. (2012, May 7). Fat Forecast: 42% of Americans Obese by 2030. *ABC News.*

Belly fat in women: Taking—and keeping—it off, http://www.mayoclinic.com/health/belly-fat/WO00128.

Whitmer RA, Gustafson DR, et al. "Central obesity and increased risk of dementia more than three decades later." *Neurology.* 2008 Sep 30;71(14):1057–64. doi: 10.1212/01.wnl.0000306313.89165.ef. Epub 2008 Mar 26.

R. Morgan Griffin, Obesity and Early Puberty: What's the Risk?, Retrieved from http://children.webmd.com/features/obesity.

Smith GI, Atherton P, Reeds DN, et al. "Dietary omega-3 fatty acid supplementation increases the rate of muscle protein synthesis in older adults: a randomized controlled trial." *Am J Clin Nutr* February 2011 vol. 93 no. 2 402–412.

Obesity and Early Puberty: What's the Risk? http://children.webmd.com/features/obesity (June, 2010).

CHAPTER 3

Schmitz KH, Lin H, Sammel MD, Gracia CR, Nelson DB, Kapoor S, DeBlasis TL, Freeman EW. "Association of physical activity with reproductive hormones: the Penn Ovarian Aging Study". *Cancer Epidemiol Biomarkers Prev,* 2007 Oct; 16(10):2042–7. Epub 2007 Sep 28.

Breast Health. (2011). *Natural Hormone Institute.* Retrieved August 26, 2012, from http://www.hormonewell.com/breastHealth_diet.html.

Exercise Lowers Estrogen Levels in Older Women, Retrieved from http://www.breastcancer.org/research-news/20100216.

Safdar A, Bourgeois JM, Ogborn DI, et al. "Endurance exercise rescues progeroid aging and induces systemic mitochondrial rejuvenation in mtDNA mutator mice". *PNAS,* (2011): 201019581, http://www.pnas.org/content/early/2011/02/18/1019581108.full.pdf+html.

Cherkas LF, Hunkin JL, Kato BS, et al. "The Association Between Physical Activity in Leisure Time and Leukocyte Telomere Length". *Arch Intern Med,* 2008; 168(2): 154–158. Doi:10.1001/archinternmed2007.39.

Padycula, J. (2012, April 18). Buddy Up for Workout. *She Knows.*

Actress goes archer: Geena Davis in Olympic archery semifinals, http://sports illustrated.cnn.com/olympics/news/1999/08/05/davis_archery_ap/ (August 1999).

After Late Start, Runner Is Speeding Through Records, http://www.nytimes.com/2012/04/02/sports/runner-kathy-martin-60-is-speeding-through-records.html?pagewanted=all (April 2012).

7 Ways Technology Helps You Lose Weight: The New Digital Diet, http://www.prevention.com/weight-loss/weight-loss-tips/7-ways-technology-helps-you-lose-weight.

CHAPTER 4

EWG Research Shows 22 Percent of All Cosmetics May Be Contaminated With Cancer-Causing Impurity, http://www.ewg.org/release/ewg-research-shows-22-percent-all-cosmetics-may-be-contaminated-cancer-causing-impurity (Feb 2007).

Exposure to Chemicals in Plastic, http://www.breastcancer.org/risk/factors/plastic (September 2012).

Braun JM, Kalkbrenner AE, et al. Impact of Early-Life Bisphenol A Exposure on Behavior and Executive Function in Children. *Pediatrics.* 2011 Nov;128(5):873–82. doi: 10.1542/peds.2011-1335. Epub 2011 Oct 24.

Kaiser Permanente Says GMO Controversy Misleading, Retrieved from http://news.health.com/2012/12/03/kaiser-permanent-says-gmo-controversy-misleading/ (December 2012).

CHAPTER 5

Risks and Benefits of Estrogen Plus Progestin in Healthy Postmenopausal Women: Principal Results From the Women's Health Initiative Randomized Controlled Trial. (2002). *Journal of the American Medical Association, 288*(3), 321–333.

Wyeth Pharmaceuticals, Inc: Prempro. (2009, May). US Food and Drug Administration. Retrieved July 23, 2012.

Winfrey, O. (2009, February). Is Hormone Replacement Therapy Right for You?. *The Oprah Show*. Retrieved July 23, 2012, from http://www.oprah.com/health/Is-Hormone-Replacement-Therapy-Right-for-You/9.

Northrup, C. (2009, January 29). Hormone Replacement Therapy Q&A Webcast. *The Oprah Winfrey Show*. Webcast retrieved from http://www.oprah.com/health/The-Hormone-Replacement-Webcast-with-Dr-Christiane-Northrup.

McGraw, R. (2009). Retrieved August 25, 2012, from http://www.robinmcgraw.com/books.html.

L. Leaseburge, Personal communications. 2011.

Renee, J. (2011, March 28). Information on the Pregnenolone Supplement. *Livestrong*. Retrieved July 23, 2012, from http://www.livestrong.com/article/408509-information-on-the-pregnenolone-supplement/.

Leonetti, H. B. (2005). Transdermal Progesterone Cream as an Alternative Progestin in Hormone Therapy. *Alternative Therapies in Health & Medicine*, *11*(6), 36–38.

Stein, D. G., Sayeed, I., & Atif, F. (2012). Progesterone Prodrugs and Analogs as Neuroprotective Agents. *Emory Institute for Drug Development*. Retrieved July 23, 2012, from http://eidd.emory.edu/progesterone-prodrugs-and-analogs.

Skelly, L., & Korschun, H. (2011, July 13). Progesterone Inhibits Growth of Neuroblastoma Cancer Cells. *Emory Woodruff Health Sciences Center*. Retrieved July 23, 2012, from http://shared.web.emory.edu/whsc/news/releases/2011/07/progesterone-inhibits-growth-of-neuroblastoma-cancer-cells-.html.

CHAPTER 6

Thompson, Holli, Your Girlfriends and Your Weight, Retrieved from http://askmissa.com/2011/12/16/your-girlfriends-and-your-weight/.

Cohen, Emma, Ejsmond-Frey, Robin, Knight, Nicola and Dunbar, R.I.M. "Rowers high: behavioural synchrony is correlated with elevated pain thresholds." Biol. Lett. Rsbl20090670. Published online September 15, 2009 doi: 10.1098/rsbl.2009.0670,http://rsbl.royalsocietypublishing.org/content/early/2009/09/14/rsbl.2009.0670.full.pdf+html.

Jaslow, R. (2012, March 27). Eating lots of chocolate helps people stay thin, study finds. *CBS News*.

Brian Buijsse, Cornelia Weikert, Dagmar Drogan, Manuela Bergmann, and Heiner Boeing. Chocolate consumption in relation to blood pressure and risk of cardiovascular disease in German adults. *European Heart Journal*, DOI: 10.1093/eurheartj/ehq068.

Hollis, J. (2012, April 16). Chew on this: study finds additional chewing reduces food intake in young adults. In Iowa State University. Retrieved from http://archive.news.iastate.edu/news/2012/apr/chewing.

5 Benefits of Properly Chewing Food. (2008). 3 Fat Chicks. Retrieved August 26, 2012, from http://www.3fatchicks.com/5-benefits-of-properly-chewing-food/.

CHAPTER 7

Discovery Health, 5 Anti-Aging Supplements That Really Work, http://health.howstuffworks.com/wellness/aging/anti-aging-tips/5-anti-aging-supplements.htm (Nov 2012).

Vadim Aksenov, Jiangang Long, Sonali Lokuge, Jane A Foster, Jiankang Liu and C David Rollo, "Dietary amelioration of locomotor, neurotransmitter and mitochondrial aging" Experimental Biology and Medicine (2010, 235): 66–76, http://ebm.rsmjournals.com/content/235/1/66.full.pdf+html.

Gahche J, Bailey R, Burt V, et al. Dietary Supplement Use Among U.S. Adults Has Increased Since NHANES III (1988–1994). NCHS data brief, no 61. Hyattsville, MD: National Center for Health Statistics. 2011.

Bailey RL, Gahche JJ, Lentino CV, et al. Dietary supplement use in the United States, 2003–2006. *J Nutr.* 2011; 141(2):261–266.

Dickinson A, Boyon N, and Shao A. Physicians and nurses use and recommend dietary supplement: report of a survey. *Nutrition Journal.* 2009; 8:29.

"11 Proven Benefits of Omega-3 Fish Oil for Women," Retrieved November 27, 2012 from http://www.ehow.com/about_5445018_proven-omega-fish-oil-women.html.

Betty Kovacs, MS, RD, "Probiotics," Retrieved November 17, 2012 from http://www.medicinenet.com/probiotics/article.htm.

"Herbal Supplements: What to Know Before You Buy," Retrieved November 17, 2012 from http://www.mayoclinic.com/health/herbal-supplements/SA00044.

"4 Dangerous (and Common) Vitamin Fillers You Must Avoid," Retrieved November 17, 2012 from http://www.draxe.com/4-dangerous-and-common-vitamin-fillers-you-must-avoid/.

CHAPTER 8

"Vitamin D Levels and oral supplementation in patients with skin cancer", *Journal of American Academy of Dermatology* Vol 62, Issue 3, Supplement 1 (March 2010): Page AB66.

Brierley Wright, "Anti-aging foods for your skin," http://www.eatingwell.com/blogs/health_blog/anti_aging_foods_for_your_skin (May 2012).

Maria Celia B Hughes, Gail M Williams, Anny Fourtanier, and Adele C Green, "Food intake, dietary patterns, and actinic keratoses of the skin: a longitudinal study", *The American Journal of Clinical Nutrition* Vol 89 no. 4, (April 2009): 1246–1255.

Peter Jaret, "Coping With Acne: Your Care Plan," Retrieved from http://www.webmd.com/skin-problems-and-treatments/acne/acne-care-11/exercise.

Robert Haas, MS, "How Chronic Insomnia Destroys Skin Health," Retrieved October 30, 2012 from http://www.lef.org.

CHAPTER 9

Vaginal Dryness, Retrieved January 13, 2013 from http://www.nlm.nih.gov/medlineplus/ency/article/000892.htm.

CHAPTER 10

Koenig, Harold G, Hays, Judith, et al, Does Religious Attendance Prolong Survival? *J Gerontol A Biol Sci Med Sci* (1999) 54 (7): M370-M376. doi: 10.1093/gerona/54.7.M370

University of Colorado at Boulder (1999, May 17). Research Shows Religion Plays a Major Role in Health, Longevity. *ScienceDaily,* Retrieved January 23, 2013, from http://www.sciencedaily.com/releases/1999/05/990517064323.htm

Koenig, H.G., Cohen H.J., George L.K., Hays J.C., Larson D.B., Blazer D.G. (1997) "Attendance at religious services, interleukin-6 and other biological indicators of immune function in older adults." *International Journal of Psychiatry in Medicine* 27 233–250

Jonas, W.B., Crawford, C.C. (2003) *Healing Intention and Energy Medicine.* New York: Churchill Livingstone.

Glazer, S. (January 14, 2005). "Can Spirituality Influence Health?" *CQ Researcher.* Vol. 15, no. 2: 1–35.

Puchalski, C., MD, (2004). Spirituality in health: the role of spirituality in critical care. *Critical Care Clinics*. Vol. 20: 487–504.

Dossey, L. MD (1993). *Healing Words*. San Francisco: Harper Collins Publishers.

General Social Surveys, 1972–2010. Conducted by the National Opinion Research Center at the University of Chicago.

CHAPTER 11

Lee, H. (2009, June). Oxytocin: The great facilitator of life. *Progress in Neurobiology*. 8(22), 127–151.

CHAPTER 12

Cohen, E. (2011, June 23). Does life online give you "popcorn brain?" *CNN*.

Be Well: Laugh. (2012). UCF Wellness and Health Promotion Services. Retrieved August 26, 2012, from http://bewellucf.com/2011/11/17/be-well-laugh/

"Is Laughter Part of Your Healthy Lifestyle?" (2012). *Healthy Living*.

Gail Larsen. (2012). "Real Speaking." Retrieved August 5, 2012, from http://www.realspeaking.com/.

Vessels, J. (2011, March 1). "Play: It's Just Good for You!" *Health & Wellness*.

CHAPTER 13

MassMutual Financial Group and Oppenheimer Funds, "From the Locker Room to the Boardroom: A Survey on Sports in the Lives of Women Business Executives," 2002.

Stephanie Wilcox, How Do Team Sports Help Develop Girls Into Future Leaders?, http://www.theglasshammer.com/news/2010/12/08/how-do-team-sports-help-develop-girls-into-future-leaders/ (December 2010).

Stevenson, Betsey. Beyond the Classroom: Using Title IX to Measure the Return to High School Sports. (Cambridge, MA: NBER Working Paper Series, National Bureau of Economic Research, 2010) , http://www.nber.org/papers/w15728.

Ernst & Young, Women Make All the Difference in the World, http://www.ey.com/GL/en/Issues/Driving-growth/Growing-Beyond—-High-Achievers—-Women-make-all-the-difference-in-the-world (2012).

Hillary Rodham Clinton, U.S. Secretary of State, announcing the Global Sports Mentoring Program, 21 June 2012.

CHAPTER 14

Parker-Pope, T. (2010, April 14). Is Marriage Good for Your Health? *The New York Times.*

Perls, Tom. New England Centenarian Study, Boston University School of Medicine, http://www.bumc.bu.edu/centenarian/overview/.

Research, Statistics, and Policy Analysis. (2012, August 2). "Social Security." Retrieved August 5, 2012, from http://www.ssa.gov/policy/docs/workingpapers/index.html.

Study: Majority of Women Becoming Primary Breadwinners. (2012, July 16). *CBS News.* Retrieved August 27, 2012, from http://washington.cbslocal.com/2012/07/16/study-majority-of-women-becoming-primary-breadwinners/.

CHAPTER 15

Excerpted from Congresswomen Linda T. Sánchez, February 25, 2010 blog. Congresswomen Sánchez represents the 39th Congressional District of California.

INDEX